the
healthy you
diet

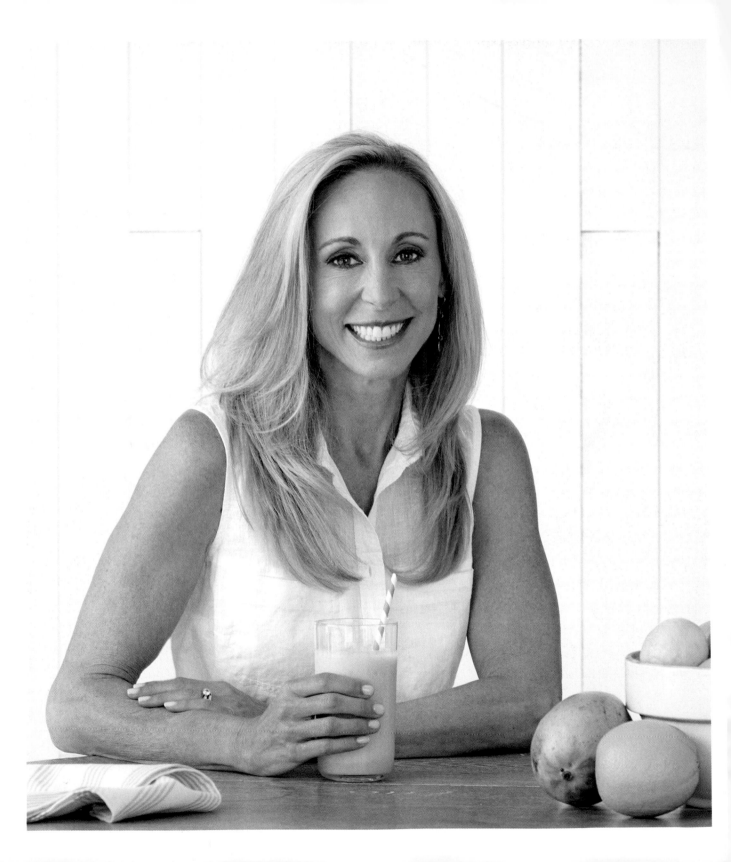

the
healthy you
diet

The 14-Day Plan
for Weight Loss with
100 Delicious Recipes
for Clean Eating

Dawna Stone

RODALE

© 2014 by Dawna Stone
Photographs © 2014 by Rodale Inc.

Rodale books may be purchased for business or promotional use or for special sales. For information, please write to:
Special Markets Department, Rodale Inc., 733 Third Avenue, New York, NY 10017

Printed in the United States of America
Rodale Inc. makes every effort to use acid-free ∞, recycled paper ♻.

Photo direction by Carol Angstadt
Photographs by Mitch Mandel/Rodale Images
Book design by Amy C. King

Library of Congress Cataloging-in-Publication Data is on file with the publisher.

ISBN 978–1–62336–549–3   hardcover

Distributed to the trade by Macmillan

2   4   6   8   10   9   7   5   3   1   hardcover

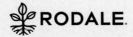

We inspire and enable people to improve their lives and the world around them.
rodalebooks.com

To my children, Kaelie and Luke,
for inspiring me to lead a healthy and passionate life;
and to my husband, Matt,
for encouraging me to always follow my dreams

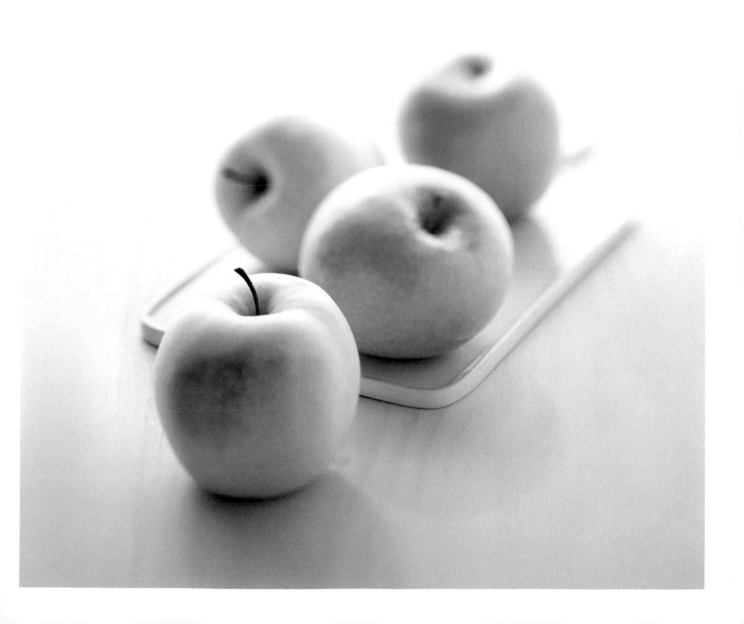

contents

part two: the healthy you recipes

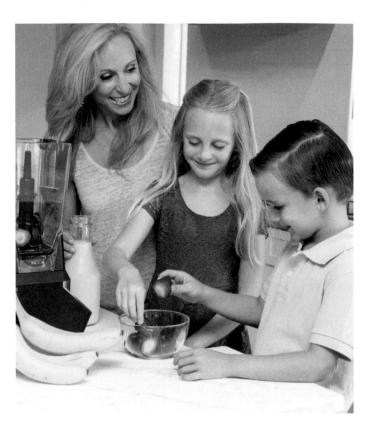

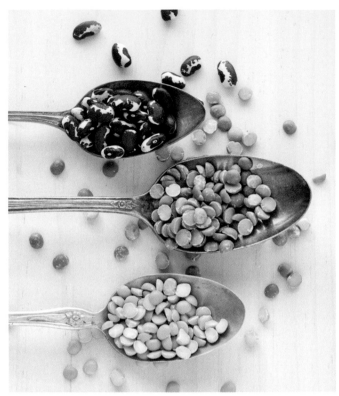

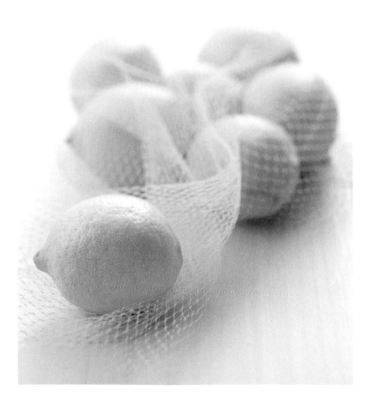

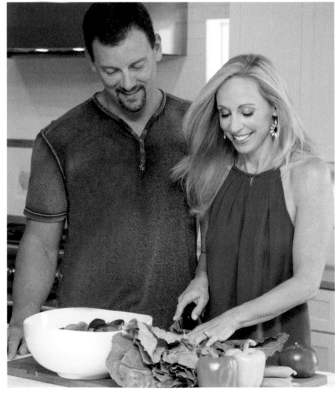

introduction

Over the past decade, I've shared my message of healthy eating and weight loss with millions. People often assume that I've always been slender and healthy, but trust me, that wasn't always the case. Just like so many others, for many years I struggled with my weight and, as a result, my health.

When I graduated from college and moved to New York City to work as a financial analyst for a Wall Street investment bank, I started to pack on the pounds. It was bad enough that I had gained (and never lost) the ubiquitous freshman 15 during my first year at school, but then, once I was out in the working world, it wasn't long before I added another 25 pounds to my frame—for a total of 40 extra pounds!

For so long, I felt that I was the only person in the world who couldn't control her obsession with food. My life was consumed by it—what to eat and when to eat. Before one meal was finished, I was thinking about the next. Because my 14-hour days were so long, I rewarded myself by grabbing unhealthy foods and snacks at the company cafeteria. After a hard day at the office, it was reassuring to know that a box of cookies waited for me at home. Some people might have been happy with a couple of cookies, but I polished off the entire package in one sitting. If there were no goodies to look forward to at home, I stopped at the corner market for some frozen yogurt and a candy bar.

I knew my eating was out of control, but none of the diets I tried helped. And believe me, I tried them all, from well-known commercial weight-loss programs to assistance at a special weight-loss clinic. At best I'd lose a few pounds, but I'd always regain them—along with a few extra.

Then one day it dawned on me that the reason I couldn't lose weight and keep it off was because the diets and programs I was using just weren't right for me! I hated getting publicly weighed in front of a roomful of strangers. I despised the tiny, tasteless, pre-packaged meals. I didn't have time to make the complicated recipes I saw in magazines and books. I loathed the eating plan designed for me by a bodybuilder—it consisted of only chicken, tuna, and vegetables. I was miserable. And I was always craving more food, because nothing satisfied me. All of those diets were useless for someone who loves food as much as I do.

In order to find a weight-loss program that worked and had everything I wanted—simple yet delicious recipes, an occasional indulgence, and options for dining out—I had to create my own. Through trial and error, I finally discovered an eating plan that worked. The weight came off quickly and easily and, most important, stayed off. I no longer craved junk food between meals or desperately shoved unhealthy foods into my mouth.

Before long, colleagues, friends, and family noticed my weight loss and asked how I did it. It seemed that everyone was just as fed up and frustrated with traditional weight-loss programs as I was. Although I never thought of what I was eating as "my plan," I was soon sharing my recipes and tips with anyone who asked, including local women's groups and clubs.

I spent the next 6 years working in the world of finance and strategy, with the exception of a 2-year stint at graduate school. It became clear that my career in the financial world limited my ability to share with others what I had discovered about eating well and losing weight. I decided to leave my job as a strategy consultant and accepted an offer to be president and general manager of a $20 million sports nutrition company. That job was my initial foray into a world that focused on health, wellness, and fitness rather than investments, banking, and management consulting. In 2001, my husband and I moved to St. Petersburg, Florida, and I became the chief marketing officer of a $700 million publicly traded company. Although it was a great company, I had become accustomed to working in an environment that inspired people to get healthy and live well. I missed helping others more than I thought I would. In 2003, I raised the money to launch a women's sports-and-fitness magazine, initially called *Her Sports* and renamed *Women's Running,* which allowed me to share what I had learned about weight loss, nutrition, and fitness with other busy women who were as desperate as I had been. As a result, I was asked to do a regular TV segment on Fox called "Healthy Living with Dawna Stone," which reached an even larger audience.

In 2006, I applied and was selected to be one of 16 contestants on *The Apprentice: Martha Stewart.* When I won the TV competition, hundreds of doors opened for me: I had my own weekly radio show. I wrote regular columns for *Body+Soul* magazine. I appeared on *Martha,* Stewart's TV show, as well as the major networks, and inspired viewers with the same healthy recipes that I had used to lose weight. I spent the next 5 years growing my magazine, launching another business, appearing on local and national TV and radio, and flying across the country to speak to large companies and organizations. In 2012, I sold both of my companies (*Women's Running* magazine and my start-up, the Women's Half Marathon running series), so I could focus on sharing my knowledge about weight loss to an even broader audience.

The Healthy You Diet is the culmination of my own experiences, as well as those of the thousands of people (you'll read some of their stories) who have successfully followed the program. The Healthy You Diet significantly changed my life, and it can change yours, too.

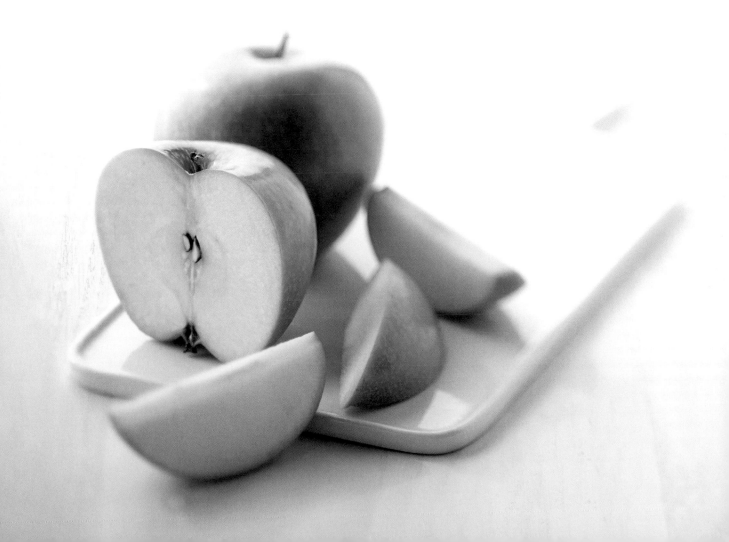

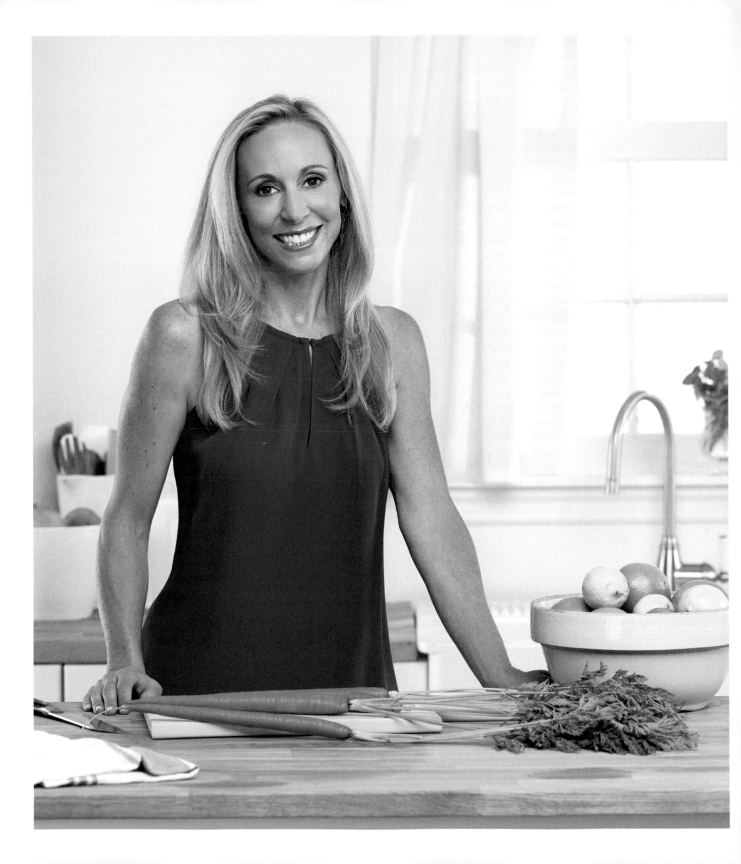

part one

a healthy you

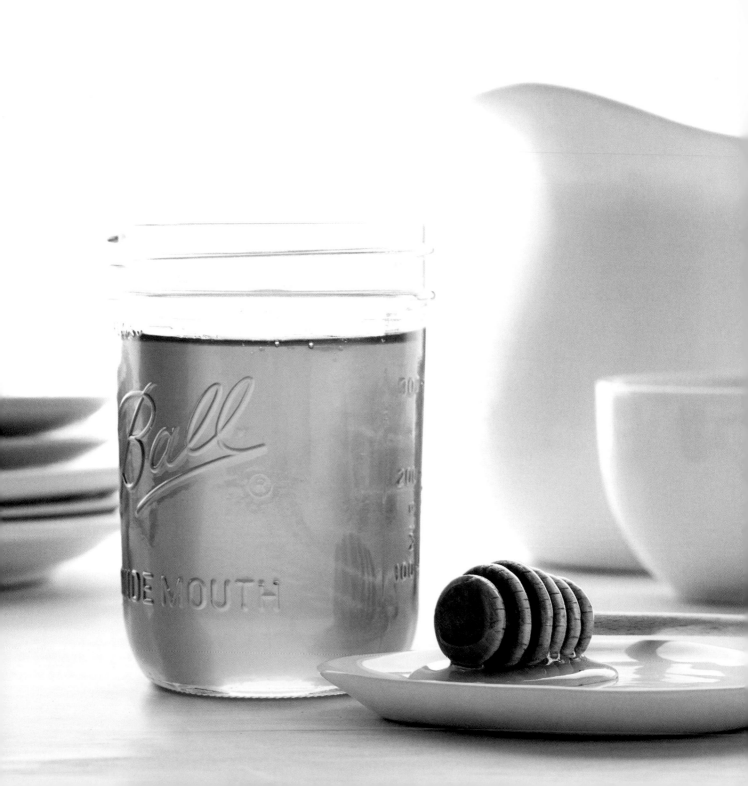

chapter

1

why choose
the healthy you diet?

One of the major reasons traditional diets don't work is that they expect
you to go cold turkey and cut certain food groups all at once. Such a drastic
change is often too much to handle, so we quickly revert back to our old eating
habits. The Healthy You Diet helps you gradually change your diet and your approach
to food.

The program is divided into two 1-week phases: the **Elimination Phase** and the
Clean Phase. During the Healthy You Elimination Phase, you'll omit one item from
what I call the Big Seven from your diet each day rather than all at once. By the end of
the week, you won't be eating or drinking sugar, wheat, dairy, processed foods, artificial
sweeteners, red meat, or alcohol. I'll explain why temporarily cutting out these foods
leads to successful weight loss and how this gradual process of elimination allows you to
adjust to changes in your diet.

During the Healthy You Clean Phase, you'll be introduced to delicious, filling recipes, all prepared without the Big Seven. For both weeks, I offer day-by-day meal plans
and easy recipes to keep you satisfied and motivated while you achieve your long-term
weight-loss goals.

The Benefits of the Healthy You Diet

While the ultimate goal of the Healthy You Diet is to help you achieve and maintain a healthy weight, it's also about discovering how you can enjoy a better life. If you're like other busy people in our fast-moving world, you may be familiar with any or all of the following symptoms:

- Lack of energy
- Trouble falling and staying asleep at night
- Feeling anxious and stressed
- Cravings for sugary and/or starchy foods; overeating
- Low self-esteem
- Digestive issues and discomfort
- Dull or lackluster skin

If you are experiencing any of those symptoms, then the Healthy You Diet is for you. It will help you lose weight as well as:

- Increase your energy levels
- Promote better sleep
- Reduce stress and anxiety
- Control food cravings and mood swings
- Raise your self-esteem
- Improve digestion
- Enhance your complexion

So much of how we feel emotionally about ourselves is tied to how we look and feel physically to others and ourselves. No matter how many pounds you're trying to lose— 10 postpregnancy or the freshman 15; perhaps 25 before your daughter's wedding or 50 to control your diabetes—the Healthy You Diet can help you lead a healthier life and achieve permanent weight loss.

Getting Started

When trying to lose weight, the most difficult step is the first one. It's so easy to convince yourself that you'll make a serious effort after the weekend or the holidays or when the new school year starts. There are hundreds of excuses for putting off your healthy-eating goals until tomorrow, next week, or next month. But before you know it, too many weekends, holidays, and school years have passed and you've done nothing—and achieved nothing.

The only thing I've found that helps people stop procrastinating and start getting healthy is to believe in the program. When I first started explaining the Healthy You Diet, the people I shared it with understood the power of the program and truly believed it would work for them—even if every other diet they tried had let them down. They believed because they saw how the Healthy You Diet worked for me. They knew it would work for them because they knew how much I love food, they saw me drink wine and eat chocolate on occasion, and they witnessed my weight loss. Seeing how easily the program worked for me gave others hope. If I could do it, so could they.

As I helped more and more people lose weight, those who were successful with the Healthy You Diet shared it with their friends. It worked for them, too. They became believers.

My dream of helping millions of people who struggle with weight loss is coming true. The Healthy You Diet now reaches people across the globe. In fact, one of our online challenges included participants from 46 states and 11 countries! As people share their accomplishments and document their successes with photographs and stories, thousands of others from all over the world are discovering the program. The "if she can do it, I can do it" attitude is contagious!

I share this with you because it's important that you believe in the program even before you start. Harboring even a little doubt can hold you back and keep you waiting until tomorrow or the day after or next week to get started and reach your goals. Take a few minutes and read some of the success stories on HealthyYouDiet.com. You'll realize that the thousands of people who have succeeded on the program—lost weight and kept it off—are just like you. If they can do it, so can you. Let's get started.

2

what kind of
eater are you?

One of the many problems with traditional weight-loss programs is that they take a one-size-fits-all approach. The truth is that we all gain and lose weight differently.

Each of us is unique, especially when it comes to eating patterns and habits. Some of us carry extra weight on our hips and butts, while others pack on the pounds around our bellies and love handles. Some of us find it easy to give up sugar and alcohol, while others think nothing of saying good-bye to red meat and artificial sweeteners but struggle to give up a nightly glass of wine and piece of chocolate. Some of us would never let a day go by without going to the gym, while for others the mere idea of exercise is frightening.

I have identified five diet personality profiles. Knowing what kind of eater you are is just as important as determining your weight-loss goals. To get the most of out of the Healthy You Diet, figure out your specific profile. Read the following descriptions, determine which one best represents you, and follow the five corresponding tips for your profile to help ensure your weight-loss success.

The Remote Controller

Do you drink coffee and eat a bagel while driving to work, inhale a sandwich while e-mailing and texting at your desk, or wolf down dinner while watching TV and folding laundry? Then you're a Remote Controller, who eats mindlessly and wonders why the pounds keep packing on.

I find that people in this category often need to lose 40 to 100 pounds. The Remote Controller knows that she needs to change her eating habits but doesn't know how or where to begin. If that sounds like you, here are some tips.

- During the 14-day Healthy You program, focus on your meal-by-meal, day-by-day progress, and stay on the Week 2 Clean Phase until you reach your goal weight.

- Eat your meals at the kitchen or dining room table. At work, find a place other than your desk to have your lunch or afternoon snack. Try a conference room, an outside table, or the steps of the building. The location doesn't matter, as long as you're not eating and working at the same time.

- Focus on each bite of food at each meal. Don't watch TV, drive, text, read, or do anything else while eating.

- Keep a food log or journal. Studies show that keeping a journal aids in weight-loss success.

- Work out at least three or four times a week. If you haven't exercised in ages or never in your life, start with a 20- to 30-minute walk, outdoors or on a treadmill. Get moving!

Before the Healthy You Diet, I was so overweight and had no idea where to begin. So far I've lost 12 pounds, I have tons of energy, and my skin has cleared up. I'm determined to stick with the Healthy You Diet.

AMBER BLACK

The Nonbeliever

If you're a Nonbeliever, you've probably just about surrendered in the battle of the bulge. Through the years, you've picked up some poor eating habits, given up on exercising, and packed on 30 to 40 pounds. You think, "Why bother? I've tried every diet in the world, and no matter what I do, I'll never fit into those skinny jeans again."

As you well know, the trouble with most diets is that they're based on deprivation. You feel fine and virtuous for the first few days on the latest fad diet, then those familiar cravings and hunger pangs move in and you're back to your old bad eating habits. Well, the Healthy You Diet is your chance to finally believe in yourself. You can be back in those skinny jeans before you know it. To reach your weight-loss goals, the Nonbeliever should:

- Stop the negative self-talk. Acknowledge your positive changes, and don't berate yourself for missteps in the past.

- Focus on eating well every day, and praise yourself for a job well done.

- Keep a food journal of what you eat and how you feel when eating. Hunger pangs and cravings are often set off by emotional issues, so look for patterns that make you want to rip open a bag of potato chips or dive into a pint of ice cream.

- Weigh yourself before you begin the program, then wait until the end of the Elimination Phase to weigh yourself again. Record the numbers in your food journal.

- Get moving, whether it means going to the gym, walking for 30 minutes a day, or taking a yoga class three times a week.

> "Before the Healthy You Diet, I was a Nonbeliever. I had just about given up on ever losing weight. But since following the diet, I have lost 16 pounds and feel 10 years younger. I've changed my relationship with food, and I'm never looking back!"
>
> Mary Heise

The Flip-Flopper

You're a Flip-Flopper if you quickly lose weight on a diet and just as quickly gain it back, along with a few additional pounds. You have great intentions but very little follow-through after the first 5 days on a diet. Your closet is filled with "fat pants" and "skinny pants," but you spend more time in the fat ones. Motivating yourself to exercise is just as difficult as sticking to a diet. Here are some recommendations for losing those extra 20 to 40 pounds:

- Set small goals, like losing 3 pounds in the next 5 days, rather than focusing on a long-term goal of losing 30 pounds. Achieving success—even through small milestones—can help the Flip-Flopper stay motivated and on track.

- Keep track of your meals in a food journal. A Flip-Flopper will often "forget" that she had a piece of cake at an office birthday party or a martini with the girls on the way home. If you make a note of everything you eat, you'll be less likely to slip off the program.

- Enlist a partner—this strategy works well for Flip-Floppers. Engage a friend, sister, or colleague to start and stay on the program with you.

- Weigh yourself before beginning the program, recording the number in your food journal, but wait until the end of the Elimination Phase to reweigh yourself. The number on the scale can fluctuate based on small factors such as clothing type, dehydration levels, and menstrual cycle, and these slight discouragements can derail the Flip-Flopper.

- Get your heart rate up and burn extra calories by running or speed walking on the treadmill, and do some resistance exercise 5 days a week.

> "I used to be a Flip-Flopper, but no more. I have tried every weight-loss program out there, from Jenny Craig to Weight Watchers to drinking shakes twice a day. I stuck with them for a week or so, and then tried eating a semihealthy diet. Even with two gym memberships, I came up with excuses not to go. Now that I've lost 9 pounds in just 14 days, I'm determined not to be the Flip-Flopper I once was. Knowing how to avoid falling into the same old bad habits has helped me stick with the Healthy You program. Eliminating certain foods was an eye-opening experience."
>
> KIM GOLDER

The Food Abuser

Do you believe that exercising regularly gives you a pass to eat whatever and whenever you want? Then you're a Food Abuser, and you can easily achieve your goals if you just take control of your diet and discard all the junk food in the house. Poor nutrition rather than a lack of exercise keeps extra pounds from coming off. Stick with the Healthy You program and those 20 to 30 pounds will disappear faster than you can say "ice cream." The following are some tips for the Food Abuser:

- Remove all junk food—cookies, ice cream, pretzels, and other unhealthy snack foods—from your kitchen for the 14 days. Out of sight, out of mouth!

- Drink water throughout the day to curb cravings. You might be thirsty rather than hungry.

- Keep track of your meals and progress in your journal.

- Limit snacks to one per day. It might be helpful to initially save your snack for after dinner rather than between lunch and dinner, because Food Abusers typically consume excess calories at night. If you like to eat in the evening or before bedtime, it's important that you break this habit. One way is to temporarily postpone your designated midafternoon snack until after dinner; then, as you get used to eating a smaller and healthier snack after dinner, you can move it back to midafternoon and completely eliminate your evening snacking habit.

- Drink a cup of herbal tea before bed or after dinner. Not only can this help you relax, but it can also deter you from nighttime nibbling.

After I read about the different kinds of eaters, it was clear that I was a Food Abuser. Giving up gluten, dairy, and sugar made a huge difference, but I also learned that maintaining portion control is an important piece of the puzzle. I guess that's why it's called Food Abuser. I also realize how much time I used to spend shopping the middle aisles, where the processed foods are at my local supermarket. Now, every time I go food shopping, I'm aware of staying on the perimeter of the store, where all the healthy choices are.

Lisa Dean

The Almost Achiever

Your goal is oh so close, but no matter what you do, you can't seem to lose those last 5 to 15 pounds. As an Almost Achiever, you lead an active lifestyle but allow yourself to eat wheat, dairy, meat, and processed and sugary foods and drink alcohol more frequently than you should. These small changes will help you reach your goal.

- Increase your water intake. When you have so few pounds to lose, staying hydrated can help control your appetite and ensure that you're eating out of hunger rather than thirst.
- Keep track of what you eat in a journal. Sometimes just being more aware of your choices is enough to help you drop those last few pounds.
- Add 15 minutes to your exercise routine.
- Focus on portion control. Cutting back on serving sizes will help you reach your ideal weight.
- Weigh yourself every day while on the 14-day Healthy You program. This will help you understand how certain food choices affect your weight. Just remember that many other variables affect the number on the scale, including water intake, dehydration, constipation, and your monthly cycle.

> *I was always just 15 pounds from my goal weight but could never quite make it to the finish line. The Healthy You Diet's challenge community gave me the positive reinforcement to stick with the program. Establishing a snack pattern rather than eating whenever I wanted to was my key to success!*
>
> LISA MARIE

Me? Like many women, I was a Food Abuser who struggled with my weight before I developed the Healthy You Diet. Once I stopped eating junk food and cut out the red meat, alcohol, dairy, and wheat, I was amazed at how quickly the pounds came off and stayed off. I still indulge on occasion, but I can now do so in moderation and without sabotaging my weight loss.

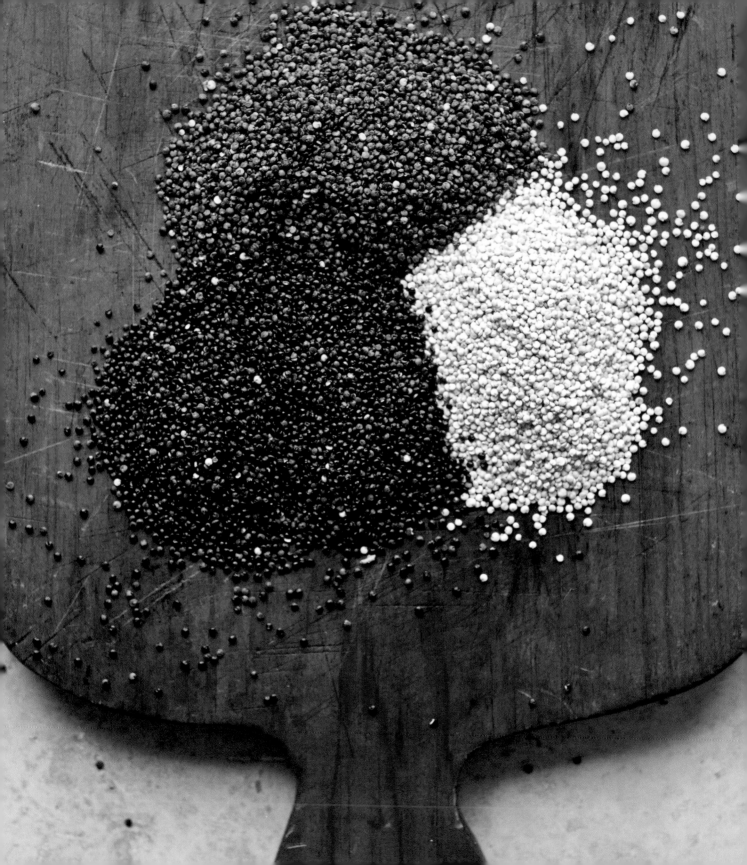

③

week 1:
the elimination phase

The Healthy You Diet consists of two 1-week phases—the Elimination Phase and the Clean Phase. These 2 weeks are designed to help you reevaluate your current food choices and eat a cleaner, healthier diet that will promote weight loss. The first phase of the Healthy You Diet, the Elimination Phase, focuses on removing one category of food each day. I call these categories the Big Seven.

The Big Seven are sugar, wheat, dairy, processed foods, artificial sweeteners (including diet soda), red meat, and alcohol. Day by day, you'll be amazed at how much better you feel and how quickly you lose weight by eliminating these foods.

Before trying the Healthy You program, people often tell me they're concerned that once they eliminate the Big Seven, there won't be enough left for them to eat. Remember, I'm asking you to eliminate these foods for just 2 weeks. It's not that I think they are necessarily "bad," but I do think that most of us make poor choices or eat these foods in excess. Temporarily eliminating them from your diet will make you more conscious of what you're eating and help you understand how they affect your mood, energy level, sleep, skin, and weight. Like the thousands of others who have lost weight—permanently—on the Healthy You Diet, you can successfully manage this phase.

Eliminating certain foods for 2 weeks will allow you to eat more healthy foods that are too often overlooked in our diets, like fresh fruits, vegetables, lean protein, certain grains, and beans. It often takes eliminating the not-so-healthy foods or those that you consume in excess to encourage you to make better choices.

I'm going to walk you through the first 7 days of the program and explain the reasons for eliminating each of the Big Seven. Knowledge is power. I've learned that when people understand why they are making changes, the process becomes easier.

DAY 1

The Process of Elimination: What, When, and Why

ELIMINATE SUGAR

For me, reducing sugar intake was the most important dietary change I made and the one that helped me lose the most weight. In addition, once I stopped eating sugar, my sense of taste became more pronounced. Eliminating sugar-laden junk food made me realize how delicious food could taste! When I stopped grabbing cookies from the break room, my blood sugar levels remained steady, and I no longer had frequent headaches or experienced those midafternoon energy highs and lows.

People often don't realize how much sugar they consume. Sugar is everywhere—in fancy coffee drinks, so-called low-fat muffins, and even fruit-flavored yogurts. In fact, the average American consumes 22 teaspoons of sugar a day! That's 16 more than the 6 teaspoons recommended for women.

Sugar is not only abundant in many everyday foods but also goes by so many other names that it can be very confusing. *Sucrose, fructose, corn syrup,* and *cane juice* are just some of sugar's aliases on the food labels of many processed products.

Sugar is also found in fruits and some vegetables, but in this case it is unprocessed, created by Mother Nature. On the program, you will be eating plenty of naturally occurring sugar to help keep any cravings under control.

When you eliminate sugary, nonnutritious foods like soda, ice cream, and candy, you'll notice immediate benefits. Your energy levels will stabilize throughout the day, you may experience fewer headaches, and overall you'll feel more in balance, with fewer mood swings.

Eliminate Sugar

BREAKFAST	LUNCH	SNACK	DINNER
Very Berry Smoothie (page 96)	Turkey and Avocado Sandwich (page 121)	1 oz low-fat string cheese and 1 medium apple	Grilled Herb Chicken (page 167), steamed broccoli, and green salad

Note: For the green salad, combine mixed greens, tomatoes, and cucumber and drizzle with ½ tablespoon Healthy You dressing of your choice (see Chapter 13).

Case Study

When 24-year-old Adrianna came to me for weight-loss advice, she insisted that she had tried everything, and even though she claimed to eat well, she couldn't lose any weight. I asked her to write down everything she ate and drank for the next 3 days.

When she returned, her journal revealed a relatively healthy diet. So why was Adrianna gaining rather than losing weight? With a little more digging, she confessed, "I guess I forgot to write down that I drink two cans of soda every day."

Together, we did the math: 165 calories per can × 2 cans per day × 365 days = 120,450 calories, or an additional 34.4 pounds of body weight per year. That's 46.5 grams of sugar per can × 2 cans per day × 365 days = 33, 945 grams, or almost 75 pounds of sugar per year!

Imagine stacking up seven 10-pound bags and one 5-pound bag of sugar. That's how much she was consuming from soda only—it didn't include the sugar in any of the other foods she ate.

Adrianna quit her soda habit cold turkey. No more sweet drinks; now she carries a refillable water bottle at all times. If she gets bored with plain water, she adds some cucumber slices and lemon or lime wedges to the bottle. As I expected, once Adrianna kicked her sugar habit, she immediately began to lose weight.

ELIMINATE WHEAT

Wheat is the most common grain consumed in the American diet, and while some grains can be good for you, most of the wheat we eat is refined and processed. As a result, many people who stop eating wheat and its by-products report that gastrointestinal problems (such as bloating, diarrhea, and constipation) and other issues (such as allergic reactions and fatigue) disappear. Most of all, they say that they quickly lose the extra pounds hanging around the middle of their bodies.

Cardiologist William Davis, MD, the author of the best-selling book *Wheat Belly,* points to eating wheat as the major reason Americans are fighting an obesity epidemic. He believes that eliminating wheat from our diets is the key to sustained weight loss and optimal health. When you cut out wheat, you will lose weight and may also find that you feel better overall. Temporarily eliminating wheat from your diet encourages you to try healthy wheat-free and gluten-free alternatives. Some of the more popular and easy-to-find wheat-free grains include amaranth, corn, millet, oats (gluten-free brands), rice, and quinoa.

Eliminating wheat can be difficult for many people. Processed wheat-based foods like frozen pizza, crackers, and pasta are convenient and inexpensive. With two small children at home, my husband and I relied on pasta as our fallback dinner at least twice a week. It is quick and easy to prepare, my kids love it, it's inexpensive, and it tastes great. I knew it would be tough for my family to stop our pasta habit, so instead, I made the simple switch from regular pasta to wheat-free types made with brown rice or quinoa. My kids didn't notice any changes, but my husband and I immediately found that we felt better—less bloated and sluggish—when we replaced our usual wheat-based pasta with wheat-free versions.

The FDA identifies wheat as one of the eight foods (along with cow's milk, eggs, peanuts, tree nuts, fish, shellfish, and soybeans) that cause 90 percent of food-related allergic reactions. More and more people are discovering that they suffer from wheat or gluten intolerances or sensitivities, which can cause headaches, weight gain, brain fog, and abdominal pain or discomfort. A wheat allergy is different from a gluten sensitivity. If you have a wheat allergy, your body might react to several different components found in wheat. (There are more than two dozen potential wheat allergens, of which gluten is just one.) Gluten intolerance, or celiac disease, occurs when the digestive system cannot tolerate gluten.

People often use the words *gluten* and *wheat* interchangeably, but gluten is not wheat. Gluten is a protein found in wheat, rye, barley, and other grains. It gives food—like bread—its chewy texture. Bread flours typically contain the highest amounts of gluten. Use the Elimination Phase as a way to determine whether a wheat-free diet works for you. If you don't notice a difference in how you feel, you can reintroduce healthy whole wheat products to your diet after the 2-week period—but *healthy* is the key term here.

Eliminate Wheat and Sugar

BREAKFAST	LUNCH	SNACK	DINNER
Oatmeal with Fresh Berries and Almond Milk (page 74)	Strawberry–Goat Cheese Salad (page 145)	5–6 oz Greek yogurt (nonfat, sugar-free) and 10 raw almonds	Chicken and Vegetable Stir-Fry (page 169)

" *After giving up sugar 2 days ago and wheat yesterday, I have noticed several positive changes. I feel wonderful! I never thought giving up wheat would make me feel better. OMG! I'm no longer constipated. I am never going to eat sugar and wheat again. My moods have improved significantly! No more mood swings. Dawna, you rock!* "

PATTY LOVE

ELIMINATE DAIRY

Like most of us, I grew up drinking milk, eating grilled cheese sandwiches, and enjoying ice cream whenever I could. My young children drink organic milk in the morning, but as they grow, I've cut back on the amount of milk they consume. I make sure they are getting adequate calcium and protein from other sources like calcium-fortified almond milk, beans, nuts, and leafy greens.

When I recall how much dairy I was eating, I'm certain that those choices directly affected my inability to lose weight. Giving up dairy during the Healthy You Diet can help you eliminate specific foods—cheese and milk—that are sabotaging your weight loss. When I first eliminated dairy, I noticed some immediate benefits. My skin cleared up, I no longer suffered from regular sinus infections, my digestive issues ceased, and I immediately lost weight. These days I consume dairy only in moderation, and when I do, I make better choices. For example, I found that checking the labels on yogurt is extremely important, as many brands are loaded with artificial sweeteners, colors, or flavors. I also look for naturally occurring sugar rather than added sugar. Some yogurts actually contain more sugar than a candy bar does!

Today there are more nondairy alternatives for milk available than ever before. Almond, soy, rice, hemp, and coconut milks are just some of the great-tasting substitutes on the market. These alternatives are also often fortified and can contain as much calcium as cow's milk. Still worried about getting enough calcium? Other excellent sources of this mineral include whole grains, beans, nuts, seeds, oranges, figs, and leafy greens like kale, broccoli, arugula, collards, and spinach—all foods that are found in abundance in the Healthy You Diet.

Eliminate Dairy, Wheat, and Sugar			
BREAKFAST	LUNCH	SNACK	DINNER
Super Green Juice (page 97)	Three-Bean Salad (page 136)	1 pear or apple	Miso-Glazed Salmon with Bok Choy (page 173)

> *Eliminating dairy was the hardest step for me because I love cheese, butter, ice cream—you name it. I didn't think I'd get past breakfast without half-and-half in my coffee and butter on my toast. But as soon as I stopped eating dairy, the weight just dropped off. I lost 6 pounds by Day 4. Another benefit is that since I gave up most dairy products (I still eat nonfat yogurt), my skin is softer and smoother, and those occasional pimples are history.*

VANESSA

ELIMINATE HIGHLY PROCESSED FOODS

Processed foods—breads, crackers, frozen foods, canned foods—were originally seen as convenient time-savers for busy families. Somewhere along the way, however, additives, preservatives, enrichments, salt, sugar, and ersatz ingredients with no nutritional value were pumped into cereals, baked goods, frozen meals, and snack foods. Research shows that for many Americans, processed foods make up the majority of their daily caloric intake, and some people spend as much as 90 percent of their food budgets on these items. No wonder America is facing type 2 diabetes and obesity crises.

So what's wrong with processed foods? The bottom line is that they contain too many empty calories and none of the vitamins, minerals, and other nutrients that our bodies need to maintain cell growth and fight diseases. When someone is diagnosed with type 2 diabetes, the first thing a doctor often tells that patient is "If you lose weight, you may not have to take insulin and constantly measure your blood sugar levels." With diabetes come related diseases, such as coronary problems and high blood pressure. Just changing what you eat and losing weight can be a big part of controlling diabetes and other illnesses.

The easiest way to drop extra pounds is to cut out processed foods and instead eat more fresh vegetables and fruits and lean proteins. Like many people with type 2 diabetes and coronary heart disease, my father was obese. About 2 years ago, he decided to try the Healthy You Diet. As a result, he lost 70 pounds in 6 months, and his doctor drastically reduced his daily insulin.

In addition, many processed foods contain astronomical amounts of sodium, which contributes to high blood pressure. But eliminating salt isn't just a matter of putting down the saltshaker. According to the Mayo Clinic, "Salt is added to make food more flavorful. Salt makes soups thicker, reduces dryness in crackers and pretzels, and increases sweetness in cakes and cookies. Salt also helps disguise a metallic or chemical aftertaste in soft drinks." So not only do we need to watch the salt we add to our food, but we also need to pay attention to how much already exists in the foods we eat.

Try to eliminate as many processed foods as you can from your diet. The freshest foods—vegetables, fruit, fish, and chicken—in the supermarket are found at the perimeter of the store. Keep that in mind and avoid the inner aisles when you shop. Or support your local farmers at markets now found in cities and towns everywhere—you'll find the freshest, just-harvested ingredients there. Yes, a dozen organic eggs will cost you more than the standard ones at the supermarket, but knowing that the producing chickens were raised on quality feed, strawberry tops, and vegetable trimmings can assure you that you're eating the best eggs you can buy. As one poster I saw says, "We pay $5 for a fancy coffee, yet aren't willing to pay the same for a dozen pastured eggs." Maybe it's time we change our priorities.

You might wonder why some of the recipes in the Healthy You Diet use canned rather than dried beans in salads, soups, and other dishes. Although dried beans are healthier, soaking and cooking them takes longer. As a busy mom and business owner, I'm often short on time, so when I cook, I usually opt for canned beans. Just make sure to select beans with little or no added sodium. It's all about the choices that are right for you.

Eliminate Highly Processed Foods, Dairy, Wheat, and Sugar

BREAKFAST	LUNCH	SNACK	DINNER
Vegetable Scramble (page 79) and Oatmeal (page 74)	Grilled Salmon and Citrus Salad (page 151)	Strawberry-Banana Smoothie (page 95)	Pasta Primavera (page 187)

> *I used to go grocery shopping once or twice a week to load up on packaged processed foods. I now go to the store more frequently to buy the freshest fruits and vegetables for my family and me. Giving up sugar and wheat was hard for me, but I lost 8 pounds on the Healthy You Challenge. Fresh foods have made such a difference in my life!*
>
> MONICA HARMES

ELIMINATE ARTIFICIAL SWEETENERS
(INCLUDING DIET SODA)

Many people believe that drinking diet beverages and eating foods with artificial sweeteners helps them in the battle against the bulge. But the opposite may be true. David Ludwig, MD, PhD, who developed the Children's Optimal Weight for Life (OWL) Program, a clinic at Boston Children's Hospital that's dedicated to the evaluation and treatment of overweight and obese children, reports that people may be more likely to replace those saved calories with other calories, ultimately offsetting any weight-loss benefits. For example, if you drink three cans of Diet Coke a day, that's a total of 3.9 calories (1.3 per can) versus 426 calories (142 per can) of Coke. Instead of thinking, "Wow, I just cut out 400 calories!" most people replace them with other unhealthy foods. How many times have you told yourself that it's okay to have that burger with fries because you ordered a low-calorie diet soda?

Dr. Ludwig also suggests that artificial sweeteners overstimulate our sugar receptors and may change how we actually taste food, thus making healthy choices like fruit and vegetables less appealing, because their flavors are subtler than those of sugary cookies, ice cream, and other sweets. We're so used to eating foods with artificial sweeteners and flavorings that we've forgotten what wholesome, clean food tastes like! We've become so used to processed foods made with artificial sweeteners that a bowl of fresh summer raspberries seems almost bland when compared with a scoop of raspberry sorbet.

Eliminate Artificial Sweeteners, Highly Processed Foods, Dairy, Wheat, and Sugar			
BREAKFAST	**LUNCH**	**SNACK**	**DINNER**
Radiant Red Juice (page 98)	Vegetarian Chili (page 118)	Sliced banana and 4–6 strawberries	Flank Steak with Arugula (page 184) and 6 oz red or white wine (optional)

Artificial sweeteners go by many names. Some of the better known are aspartame (trade names: Equal and NutraSweet), saccharin (Sugar Twin and Sweet'N Low), and sucralose (Splenda). And although some sweeteners, like stevia-based ones (Truvia), are called natural, they are often chemically processed when made into powder form.

Most of the recipes in the Healthy You Diet are sugar free. When a touch of sweetness is needed, I typically use honey or agave nectar.

Case Study

Grace drank a six-pack of caffeinated diet cola every single day. She downed the first can in her car on the way to work to get herself up and running for the day. While her coworkers brought cups of tea or coffee to morning meetings, you could count on Grace to be sipping on a can of cola. She had two more at lunchtime and midafternoon. She drank still another with dinner and had her last soda of the day before bed. And here's the thing: Despite drinking all that sugar-free soda, Grace couldn't lose a single pound.

When we looked at Grace's 3-day food diary together, it wasn't surprising that she couldn't lose weight. For breakfast, she ate a sugary muffin (with her first soda). More often than not, a colleague brought a box of doughnuts to morning meetings, and Grace indulged. With two slices of pizza for lunch, Grace was consuming nearly 1,700 calories, just shy of the daily total recommended for a woman—and the day was only half over. I explained to Grace that she was sabotaging her weight-loss efforts by thinking that as long as she drank low-calorie soda, she could eat whatever she wanted.

Stopping cold turkey wasn't going to work for Grace, so she slowly cut back over a 2-week period. Because her taste buds were so zapped, she found it difficult and boring to drink plain water. I suggested that she add an orange slice, a lemon slice, and some cucumber chunks to her water bottle and take it with her everywhere. Once Grace kicked the diet soda habit, she no longer craved early morning sweets. "Once I eliminated sugar and artificial sweeteners from my diet, I couldn't believe how much better simple food tastes," she says. "These days breakfast is a fresh juice smoothie or scrambled eggs, lunch is fish tacos or three-bean chili, and dinner is grilled salmon or chicken with steamed vegetables and quinoa. The best part is that I lost 18 pounds in just 2 months!"

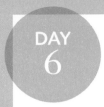

DAY 6

ELIMINATE RED MEAT

We are a nation of red-meat eaters. (To me, red meat includes any cuts of beef, veal, lamb, pork, and game.) Steak houses, where a 12- to 16-ounce steak is the norm, are often the go-to choice for dining out. When you invite people to your home during the summer, chances are good that you'll serve burgers, steaks, or hot dogs from the grill. During the winter, comfort foods like meat-based stews and chilis take center stage. Low-carb and Paleo diets have made red meat more in demand than ever. Americans still eat large quantities of red meat despite studies that show that eliminating it from the diet is one of the keys to disease-free health and longevity.

The upside of eating red meat is that it contains protein (essential for muscle growth), vitamin B_{12}, and iron. Let's face it, red meat tastes good, but too often we choose fatty cuts (prime rib, spareribs, and sausages) over lean (sirloin, pork tenderloin, and top sirloin) and portion sizes that are just too large for today's sedentary lifestyle.

For the Elimination Phase on the Healthy You program, you'll cut out red meat toward the end of Week 1 and for all of Week 2. Some people report that once they give up red meat, they feel better for no specific reason. Should you decide to reintroduce red meat into your diet, eat a lean cut like flank steak or filet mignon just once a week. Keep the serving size to 3 to 4 ounces for women and 4 to 6 ounces for men.

I still enjoy eating a petite filet about once a month. Even when I order a small steak, I usually bring home the leftovers in a doggie bag for my pup. Three to 4 ounces of perfectly cooked filet is just enough to satisfy my craving for red meat without derailing my healthy eating habits.

Eliminate Red Meat, Artificial Sweeteners, Highly Processed Foods, Dairy, Wheat, and Sugar			
BREAKFAST	**LUNCH**	**SNACK**	**DINNER**
Vegetable Omelet (page 78) and 1 slice melon	Pasta Salad with Vegetables (page 138)	1 apple and 1 Tbsp natural peanut butter	Halibut with Tomato-Mango Salsa (page 179), quinoa, steamed asparagus, and 6 oz red or white wine (optional)

" *I confess that I was eating red meat three or four times a week, so it was the hardest thing for me to give up. I find that I'm much more focused since giving up red meat—and I lost 5 pounds in just 2 weeks.* "

KELLY KEANE

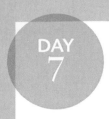
DAY
7

ELIMINATE ALCOHOL

According to Betty Kovacs, director of nutrition for the New York Obesity Nutrition Research Center Weight Loss Program, drinking alcohol can cause you to eat more and, as a result, gain weight. Research shows that people ingest 20 percent more calories when alcohol is consumed before a meal and 33 percent more if you include the alcohol's calories, too.

We often associate only food with calories and forget that beverages can contain a lot. Calories from alcohol quickly add up, especially when mixed drinks are on the menu. For example, a margarita can have as many as 550 calories; a piña colada, 586; and a mai tai, 620! When watching your weight, it's best to skip the fancy drinks and stick to beer, wine, or drinks made with noncaloric mixes like club soda.

Although I admittedly enjoy a cocktail on the weekends or the occasional nice glass of wine over dinner with my husband, it is undeniable that eliminating or reducing alcohol makes the weight-loss process much easier.

If you're trying to lose weight, think before you drink. Many people find that giving up alcohol is the secret to successful and permanent weight loss. Once you reach your desired weight, you can slowly reintroduce alcohol into your diet. Save those cocktail calories for weekends and special occasions.

Eliminate Alcohol, Red Meat, Artificial Sweeteners, Highly Processed Foods, Dairy, Wheat, and Sugar

BREAKFAST	LUNCH	SNACK	DINNER
Spinach, Tomato, and Basil Frittata (page 77) or Vegetable Omelet (page 78) and ½ cup fresh fruit	Quinoa, Cranberry, and Almond Salad (page 139)	Hummus with Vegetables (page 201)	Chicken Tacos (page 172)

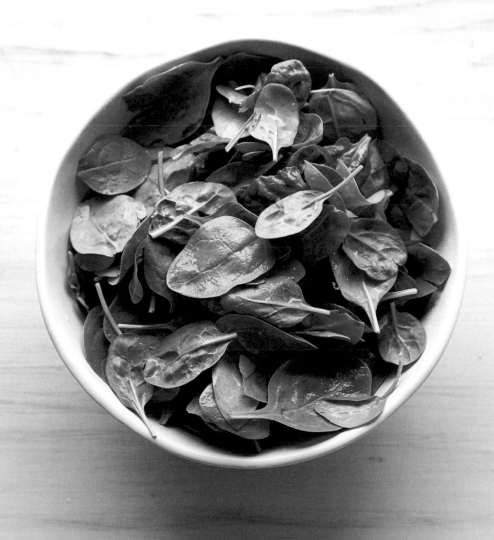

"My husband and I spend time every weekend at our camper. After a long day outdoors, we like to sit back and have a couple of beers, so giving up alcohol was difficult. But the results—8 pounds lost in 2 weeks—were amazing. Plus, I have so much more energy, and my clothes fit better."

Sylvia Smith

week 2:
the clean phase

The Clean Phase is a 7-day continuation of the final day of the Elimination Phase. During the Clean Phase, you will continue to eat a diet free of sugar, wheat, dairy, processed foods, artificial sweeteners, red meat, and alcohol.

Like the Elimination Phase, the Clean Phase is temporary. During the Clean Phase, your body will feel lighter and more energetic, your mind will be clearer and more focused, and your sleep will be deeper and more restful. The results you see will keep you on track and determined to follow the Healthy You Diet.

The Clean Phase focuses on nourishing your body. During this week, you will eat foods that are fresh, wholesome, and nutrient rich, as well as free of artificial ingredients, additives, and preservatives. You'll enjoy eating fruits, vegetables, shellfish, fish, nuts, seeds, and legumes that may be unfamiliar to you.

Following both the Elimination Phase and the Clean Phase is essential if you want to see results from the Healthy You Diet. These eye-opening 2 weeks will show you how what you've been habitually eating has been sabotaging your weight-loss efforts, especially if many of those foods are processed and contain empty calories.

The Clean Phase will change how you think about food forever. Once you discover that you don't want or need those unhealthy or nutritionally empty foods and how much better you feel without them, you'll become a knowledgeable and more mindful eater. When you go out for drinks with your girlfriends, you'll pass on the pretzels and other bar snacks. Maybe you'll order a glass of wine instead of a sugary cocktail. On business trips, you'll find yourself ordering oatmeal and fresh fruit for breakfast instead of piling a plate with muffins, French toast, and pancakes from the hotel's breakfast buffet. When dining out with your family at your favorite Mexican restaurant, you'll choose chicken and vegetable fajitas without the tortillas in place of cheese enchiladas. You'll be amazed how in just 2 weeks, you can change your entire outlook on food.

The following meal plans will help you choose what to eat for breakfast, lunch, dinner, and a snack for the next week. You can follow the program as written, or feel free to substitute one meal for another. If you'd rather have Wild Rice–Spinach Soup (page 104) for lunch on Day 11, then enjoy Spinach, Pear, and Walnut Salad (page 157) on Day 13 instead. If there's a meal you don't like or can't eat, then remove it from the plan entirely and enjoy a meal from another day. For instance, if you're allergic to shellfish, substitute Day 8's Crab Cakes (page 195) with Day 11's Fish Tacos with Mango-Avocado Salsa (page 180).

Thousands of people have already found success on the program. Although substitutions are allowed, especially if you're allergic to or dislike a particular food, following the program as closely as possible will help ensure your success, too.

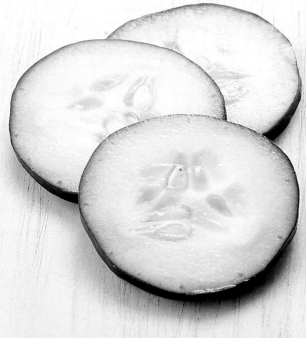

DAY 8

BREAKFAST
Super Green Juice (page 97)

LUNCH
Red Quinoa Salad with Black Beans and Avocado (page 141)

SNACK
Fresh Salsa and Tortilla Chips (page 204)

DINNER
Crab Cakes (page 195) and steamed green beans

DAY 9

BREAKFAST
Pineapple-Avocado Smoothie (page 91)

LUNCH
Vegetable Soup (page 113) and green salad

SNACK
Celery sticks and 1 tablespoon natural peanut butter

DINNER
Black Bean Tostadas with Salsa (page 197)

Note: For the green salad, combine mixed greens, tomatoes, and cucumber and drizzle with ½ tablespoon Healthy You dressing of your choice (see Chapter 13).

DAY 10

BREAKFAST
Strawberry-Banana Smoothie (page 95)

LUNCH
Lentil-Carrot Salad (page 137)

SNACK
1 cup red or green grapes

DINNER
Rosemary Chicken and Wild Rice (page 166)

DAY 11

BREAKFAST
Vegetable Scramble (page 79) and Oatmeal (page 74)

LUNCH
Spinach, Pear, and Walnut Salad (page 157)

SNACK
Magic Mango Smoothie (page 90)

DINNER
Fish Tacos with Mango-Avocado Salsa (page 180)

DAY 12

BREAKFAST
Radiant Red Juice (page 98)

LUNCH
Chicken and Brussels Sprouts Slaw (page 148)

SNACK
1 apple and 10 raw almonds

DINNER
Seared Scallops and Succotash (page 183)

DAY 13

BREAKFAST
Vegetable Omelet (page 78) and 1 cup fresh fruit

LUNCH
Wild Rice–Spinach Soup (page 104)

SNACK
Hummus with Vegetables (page 201)

DINNER
Chicken Skewers with Honey-Lime-Chile Sauce (page 171) and green salad

Note: For the green salad, combine mixed greens, tomatoes, and cucumber and drizzle with ½ tablespoon Healthy You dressing of your choice (see Chapter 13).

DAY 14

BREAKFAST
Super Green Juice (page 97)

LUNCH
Crab, Mango, and Avocado Stacks (page 152)

SNACK
1 apple or pear

DINNER
Snapper and Asparagus en Papillote (page 174) and brown basmati rice

5

frequently asked questions

When I speak to individuals or groups and share the Healthy You Diet, these are the questions (with answers) that I'm most often asked.

What do you mean by "clean eating"?

Clean eating means different things to different people. To me, it means eating food in its natural state or as close to that as possible. That means food that is free of artificial flavors, colors, sweeteners, preservatives, hormones, and antibiotics and is unprocessed and, whenever possible, organic. On the Healthy You Diet, clean eating also means eliminating those foods that can sabotage your weight-loss efforts and health—sugar, wheat, dairy, highly processed foods, artificial sweeteners, red meat, and alcohol.

When it comes to clean eating, however, I'm realistic. I try to eat clean as often as possible, but I also believe in indulging in moderation. Life without chocolate, cookies, wine, and ice cream wouldn't be much fun. I eat clean most of the time so I don't have to feel guilty when I do occasionally indulge. That said, even when I do indulge, I find myself paying close attention to the food labels.

Why are foods eliminated in the suggested order?

When attempting to clean up your diet, eliminating sugar, wheat, and dairy can have a huge and often nearly immediate impact on how you feel. However, it can be daunting and difficult for many people to eliminate these three food groups, so I wanted them to be the first to go, while everyone's enthusiasm, willpower, and dedication to the program are the strongest. In just a few short days, you will notice positive changes in your energy levels, sleep patterns, hunger, and cravings, which should keep you motivated to stay on the program.

How much weight can I expect to lose?

Participants have lost anywhere from 6 to 14 pounds during the 14-day Healthy You Diet by eating a healthier, cleaner diet and eliminating the food categories that are known to sabotage weight loss.

Every time I try to lose weight, I have a hard time staying motivated. I can follow a program for a few days, but then I find myself reverting back to my old habits. Do you have any advice that will help me stay focused and be successful?

First, most diets insist that you immediately give up all of your favorite foods. The Healthy You Diet eliminates one food group every day, so you don't go cold turkey. This makes it much easier to stay with the program. If you're looking for support and motivation to reach your weight-loss goals, join the free 14-day challenge at dawnastone.com/healthyyouchallenge.

Can I drink coffee or tea during the 14-day Healthy You Diet?

Yes, you can drink coffee and tea during the Elimination Phase and Clean Phase. Instead of animal-based milk, add a splash of unsweetened almond milk. Avoid all creamers.

Can I add artificial sweetener to my coffee or tea?

All artificial sweeteners (Splenda, Equal, Sweet'N Low, etc.) are eliminated on Day 5 of the Healthy You program. You may wonder if stevia, an intensely sweet herb that has been used as a sweetener in its natural form for centuries, is allowed. It is often found in powder form under the brand name Truvia, and I treat this processed stevia like any other artificial sweetener and eliminate it during the program.

If you frequently consume artificial sweeteners (including diet sodas), you might have a headache for a day or two when you eliminate them, but you'll soon notice that you feel better and have more energy.

If, after the 14-day program, you find that you still miss sweetened coffee or tea, try adding a small amount of a more natural sweetener like honey or agave. You might, however, be amazed at how much better your food tastes when it's no longer masked by artificial flavors.

What should I drink instead of diet sodas and sweet beverages?

It's important to keep yourself hydrated throughout the day, so I always have a bottle of water or unsweetened iced tea on my desk or in my car. I often add a slice of lemon, lime, or orange to my water. Or try adding a few cucumber slices and mint leaves—it makes you feel like you're at a spa. You can also try some of the many herbal teas available, and enjoy them hot or chilled.

There are a few juices included in the 14-day meal plan. Since I don't own a juice extractor, can I use a blender instead?

Blenders and juicers yield different quantities. If you don't have a juicer, then choose one of the smoothies instead, or select another breakfast recipe, making sure it adheres to whatever foods are eliminated for that day.

Can I add protein powder to my morning smoothies?

If protein powder isn't included in specific breakfast drinks, such as Super Green Juice (page 97) or Pineapple-Avocado Smoothie (page 91), then steer clear of it for the 14 days. Protein powders are processed and often contain additives and preservatives. You will be eating plenty of protein at your meals.

Since I'm a vegetarian, how can I participate in the 14-day program?

Although the meal plans do include meat and seafood, don't let that deter you. The program was meant to be flexible, and you can easily alter it to work with a vegetarian diet. For example, if a meat or seafood dish is listed for dinner, feel free to substitute it with Vegetarian Chili (page 118), Nori Rolls with Avocado-Wasabi Sauce (page 129), or Roasted Vegetable Pasta (page 188). If you find a favorite vegetarian recipe, double it and store as directed so you have extra for lunches and dinners. As long as you follow the program instructions for what food item is eliminated each day, you can plan your recipes accordingly.

What do you recommend if I exercise regularly?

If your workout lasts 45 minutes or more and is moderately intense to very intense, you may need some additional calories. I suggest trying to stick to the foods in the program and just add another snack, such as a piece of fruit or a small handful of almonds, after your workout. You can pick a snack from another day, as long as it adheres to the program. For example, don't eat yogurt once dairy is eliminated.

Is it okay to have leftovers from dinner or lunch the next day?

Absolutely! I do it all the time. I often double one of my favorite dinner recipes, like Vegetarian Chili (page 118), so I can enjoy it 2 days in a row.

The goal of the Healthy You Diet is to eliminate the foods that get in the way of permanent weight loss. I don't want you to become bogged down because you don't have time to make a meal—that's one of the many reasons traditional diets are so unsuccessful. We all have busy lives and schedules, so there is no one-size-fits-all diet. Whether you're sticking to the plan exactly or making extra servings and having leftovers the next day, simply eliminating the Big Seven and eating clean will have those excess pounds dropping off.

What if I'm not hungry?

I do not suggest skipping any meals. Eating at regular intervals is important for keeping your blood sugar and energy levels up and ensures that you stay motivated on the program. Surprisingly, skipping meals may not help you lose more weight. In fact, having too few calories during the day could actually hinder your weight loss by triggering nighttime eating. A study published in the *Journal of the American Medical Association* found that people with night eating syndrome—in which people consume the majority of their food late at night—often eat only a third of their daily calories by 6 p.m., while people who don't eat at night typically consume three-quarters of their food by that time. If it's noon and you find you're not hungry, then go ahead and wait an hour for lunch, but don't skip it.

If I miss my afternoon snack, can I eat it after dinner, or should I skip it for that day?

Your afternoon snack will keep your energy levels up and control hunger, so make an effort to eat it every day. If you have to miss it in the afternoon, then enjoy it after dinner rather than skipping it.

Since I don't like beans, can I substitute another food?

I encourage you to at least give a few of the bean recipes a try. If you still don't like them, then you can substitute a meal from another day instead of including foods that are not part of the meal plan. This is also true if you are allergic to any of the foods on the program, such as shellfish, or don't like a particular food—you can just select a meal from another day.

I followed the Healthy You Diet for 14 days with some friends. I lost several pounds, but they all lost more weight and faster. What did I do wrong?

We're all individuals with our own metabolisms and bodies. That's what makes each of us unique. Everyone loses and gains weight at different rates and in different areas of their bodies. You may lose slowly in the beginning, and then see a sudden surge toward the end of the program. Don't become discouraged. If you stick to the program and give it time, you will see significant changes.

What immediate changes will I notice on the Healthy You Diet?

Once you eliminate sugar and artificial sweeteners from your diet, you may experience headaches, but that is common when starting any clean eating program. Stay strong and keep with the program! By Day 4, you'll notice that your energy levels are higher, and you'll experience fewer midafternoon crashes and cravings. The lethargy that often follows big meals will disappear, and soon you'll feel great all the time.

I had great results—I lost 10 pounds!—during the 14-day program, but I seem to have reached a plateau. How can I continue losing weight?

Be patient and realize that this is all part of the process. Even with solid determination and hard work, you can go from losing weight to staying at your new weight for a short period of time. Push forward and you will continue to drop pounds after your body's metabolism resets itself to your lower weight. Know that if you stick with the Healthy You Diet, your body will definitely respond to the positive changes you're making. By anticipating some bumps in the road, you'll be better equipped to stay positive so you can reach your ultimate weight-loss goals.

Since I eat a fairly clean diet with lots of fruits and vegetables, can I skip the Elimination Phase and go right to the Clean Phase?

It depends on what you mean by "fairly clean." Even if you're eating what is considered a healthy diet, you may not be aware that many foods are highly processed and contain sugar, wheat, and dairy. To be successful with the Healthy You Diet, start with the Elimination Phase. If, however, you are already wheat or dairy free, you can select a wheat- or dairy-free alternative during the first few days of the program.

long-term success

The Healthy You Diet isn't a fad diet. It doesn't make promises that go unfulfilled. If you follow the program, you will lose weight, as attested to by the thousands of people who have successfully done so. Yes, I want you to lose weight, but most of all, I want you to alter permanently how you look at the food you eat. My philosophy is rooted in being kind to your body and fueling it with meals that are healthy and wholesome. If you adhere to my philosophy, you will lose weight.

If you're like me, then I'll bet that you have your favorite indulgences—a slice of pizza, an ice cream cone, or a chocolate bar. It's difficult if not impossible to even think about giving up these treats forever. The knowledge of not being able to eat something makes that food suddenly even more desirable and appealing. Tell me I can't have that piece of chocolate and all I can think about is how much I want it! I find it completely unrealistic to tell someone who loves pizza, cookies, or other favorites that she can never eat them again. The objective of the Healthy You program is to encourage you to eat a cleaner diet and provide you with the tools you need to make better selections when it comes to food choices.

Complete deprivation of our favorite comfort foods is another reason that traditional diets fail. Every diet that I tried and failed at featured a long list of off-limits foods, such as chocolate, pizza, and alcohol. For some reason, even if I never craved something before starting the diet, I desperately wanted to eat it once it was forbidden forever. As a result, my best attempts at following the diet were sabotaged.

Knowing that you can incorporate some of your favorite foods into your diet after the first 2 weeks on the Healthy You program gives you the incentive to persevere. The secret to indulging while losing weight or maintaining weight loss is to indulge once a week. Food is meant to be savored and enjoyed. Always denying yourself a great restaurant meal or two scoops of ice cream will make you resentful and less likely to stay with the program. Enjoying a once-a-week exception after you complete the 14-day plan will keep you on track and not feeling deprived.

Another interesting aspect of a once-a-week indulgence is that it may bring back that heavy, lethargic feeling or lack of clarity you experienced back when you were consuming wheat, sugar, dairy, processed foods, red meat, and alcohol. You may find that you no longer desire these foods in excess.

> ❝I've suffered with digestive issues for many years. I turned to the Healthy You Diet to see if a clean-eating program might help. After just 14 days, there were significant changes in how I felt—no more stomach discomfort after eating. As I slowly incorporated wheat back into my diet, my digestive problems returned, and I quickly realized that eating wheat products just wasn't worth the indulgence. I'm so thankful for this program, because it helped me pinpoint what was causing my abdominal pain. No more wheat for me! ❞
>
> JOSH MADDEN

Something that helped me was picking 1 day a week to indulge—a day that never fluctuates regardless of my schedule. It gave me motivation to eat clean, healthy food the rest of the week.

For more than 15 years, I've been able to stay within 3 or 4 pounds of my goal weight by eating clean most of the time and indulging on occasion. I can maintain my goal weight as long as I stick to the Healthy You program and enjoy my treats at one meal.

My indulgence day—usually Saturday—looks something like this.

BREAKFAST

Two-egg omelet with tomato, onion, and spinach and small fresh-fruit salad

LUNCH

Large salad with grilled fish or chicken

SNACK

Hummus and fresh vegetables

INDULGENT DINNER

Margarita flatbread pizza

Glass of wine

Since most of us do our socializing and eating on the weekends, I recommend choosing Saturday or Sunday as your regular indulgence day. Those who pick a weekday often find that they want to indulge again when the weekend rolls around. Pick 1 day and stick to it. If your regular indulgence day is Saturday but you're invited to a party on Friday, don't switch your indulgence day. Make healthy choices at the party, knowing that you can indulge in your favorite treat the next day.

Allowing yourself to indulge without guilt in your not-so-healthy foods works only in moderation. On your indulgence day, select one meal or snack to eat your favorite food and keep the rest of the day's meals clean. If you crave pancakes for breakfast, enjoy them, but then be sure to eat a healthy lunch, dinner, and snack for the remainder of the day. If you plan to have pizza for dinner, then make sure your breakfast, lunch, and snack are on the Healthy You program. If you've been thinking about a piece of double chocolate cheesecake all week, go for it, knowing that your other meals for the day are free of sugar, wheat, and dairy.

The Healthy You Diet doesn't condone an all-you-can-eat splurge. Even though you can have any food you want (and I mean anything), you need to watch your portions. That means two slices of pizza, not the entire pie; one slice of chocolate cake, not two (or more). Enjoy a 4-ounce filet, not a 16-ounce porterhouse steak. If you stick with a normal rather than supersize serving of your favorite indulgence, you can still lose weight.

If you don't want to indulge once a week, then you don't have to. The choice is yours. For me, having a few treats sufficiently satisfies my cravings until the next week.

Before I created the Healthy You program, I suffered from what I call postindulgence guilt. In fact, while living in New York, I walked by the same bakery twice a day. In the window were the largest cupcakes I had ever seen—actually, they were the size of cakes. I often stopped to admire them, like a pair of expensive shoes I couldn't afford. I just couldn't get those ginormous cupcakes out of my mind, so one day, I entered the bakery and bought the biggest chocolate cupcake topped with a thick, rich swirl of buttercream icing.

Within minutes of leaving the bakery, I devoured the entire thing. It tasted even better than it looked! As soon as I licked the last bit of icing from my fingers, I began to feel guilty. In those days, such postindulgence guilt sent me spiraling into a multiday, bad-food binge. Since I had already done some damage to my dieting determination, I figured, why not give in completely? On the days that followed my cupcake episode, I ate chocolate, cookies, and a pint of mint-chocolate-chip ice cream.

Once I created the Healthy You program, I accepted that it's possible and necessary to enjoy indulgences every once in a while. Instead of slipping into a guilt-ridden junk-food fest for one, I encourage myself to enjoy a treat now and then. These indulgences now motivate me to make my next meals as healthy as possible.

At speaking engagements, I often tell this story about reaching the realization that a once-a-week indulgence is actually a positive thing, and people come up to me and share their own quirky eating tales. No matter how hard we try, none of us can be perfect when it comes to eating healthy all the time. So give yourself a break, and don't beat yourself up. Indulge in that ice cream cone, some french fries, or a giant cupcake, as long as you're eating a healthy, clean diet most of the time.

This approach is what makes the Healthy You program doable and sustainable. The first 2 weeks provide you with the foundation for clean, healthy eating. Then, by eating a mostly clean diet and indulging once a week, you no longer feel deprived or like a prisoner chained to a hopeless diet.

What happens after you finish the 2-week program is entirely up to you. People who follow the program as outlined typically lose between 6 and 14 pounds during the 14 days. If you want to lose more weight, then stay on the Clean Phase for longer than a week. Whether you choose to continue eating clean after the 2-week period or reintroduce some of the eliminated foods, I suggest that you still include a day and a meal when you can enjoy a favorite food without guilt.

> *I'm not a big red-meat or processed-foods eater, but I love bread. I never thought I could give up sandwiches until I did the Healthy You Diet. I honestly don't even think about eating bread now, because brown rice and quinoa satisfy my carb cravings. I also knew I had to give up artificially sweetened diet beverages (I was a Crystal Light addict!), and the Healthy You Diet helped me do it. I am continuing on with the program to see what more I can accomplish. Things I miss? A glass of wine will be my 'indulgence' this weekend, and I often think about eating some Greek yogurt or cheese, which I can now do in moderation.*
>
> AMY STIFF

I understand that for some people, it seems counterintuitive to promote clean eating and then suggest an occasional splurge, but as I mentioned earlier, I don't think any food should be restricted all the time. By freely allowing yourself to indulge once a week, you remove the guilt that threatens to sabotage your attempts to lose weight.

So yes, you can have your pizza, cake, or ice cream and eat it, too—just as long as you make smart choices at other meals and don't polish off the entire pizza, cake, or pint of ice cream.

chapter

real-life challenges

There are times and occasions when it can be difficult to eat clean and maintain your weight-loss achievements and goals. Attending work events 4 nights in a row, traveling for business or pleasure, or celebrating the holidays with family and friends can challenge your determination. It's easy to stick with a program if you're preparing your meals in your own home, but once you step outside your comfort zone, there are many temptations to push you off track.

I've learned that if I plan ahead, I won't be surprised or faced with temptations.

Pack Healthy Meals and Snacks

A delayed or canceled flight, which is so common these days, is enough to make anyone want to rip into junk food while stuck in an airport terminal. When traveling on a long flight—say, coast-to-coast—take along any of the Healthy You salads with a small container of dressing (no more than 3.4 ounces, per Transportation Security Administration regulations). If you're taking a long road trip, picnic with your own nutritious food— fresh fruit, nuts, cut-up vegetables, and a small container of hummus or other dip— instead of pulling into the fast-food restaurants, full of unhealthy choices, that dot the interstate highways. If you're facing a busy week at the office, make sure you have some fresh fruit on your desk to appease that afternoon sweet tooth. If the snack bar at your kids' baseball or soccer games beckons, having a healthy option in your car will keep you satisfied.

Dining Out

Whether meeting friends for dinner or taking the family out to celebrate good report cards or a happy milestone, going out to eat is a large part of our social lives. Dining out is fun and gives everyone the opportunity to try new foods. When it comes to choosing restaurants, plan ahead so you can maintain your goals.

Almost every restaurant now posts its menu online, so you can decide what you're going to order even before you leave home. By narrowing your options ahead of time, you won't be tempted by unhealthy offerings or worried that the restaurant doesn't have something that you can enjoy.

Today's restaurants offer many choices. You can order grilled chicken without the sauce, roasted fish with a choice of vegetables, or a salad topped with grilled shrimp. If everyone wants Italian food, that's no problem. Just avoid the bread basket and the creamy sauces. Order a bowl of soup and ask for a double order of salad with dressing on the side. Going Mexican? Ask for a bowl of black bean soup and chicken and vegetable fajitas without the tortillas.

When dining out, feel free to tell the server that you want your dressing or any sauce served on the side. Ask for brown rice, a plain baked potato, or a sweet potato instead of french fries. Explain that you would like your vegetables steamed rather than sautéed. Restaurants are in the hospitality business, and that means making you feel welcome and eager to return to establishments that are willing to accommodate your needs.

Try to avoid all-you-can-eat buffets. It's almost impossible to show restraint in the presence of so many choices. If you attend meetings and conferences with large groups, you may encounter buffet tables set up for breakfast, lunch, and dinner. Walk around the table and make a mental note of what you can and can't eat, then pick up a plate and fill it with wise choices. At these same professional events, pass on the cookies, bagels, and pastries set out on tables outside meeting rooms. Enjoy a piece of fruit if you're hungry, but I find that most people eat from these snack tables out of boredom rather than hunger.

Snacks

Somewhere along the food chain, *snacks* became synonymous with *poor eating habits,* but healthy snacks are essential to a successful weight-loss program. Since it's difficult to go without eating something for an extended length of time (except while sleeping at night, when your brain and body fast, rest, and regenerate), the secret is to choose the right snack to enjoy midafternoon. I find that one-quarter cup of almonds, some hummus with sliced vegetables, or a piece of fruit takes the edge off my afternoon hunger. As always, be sure to read the nutrition labels on snack foods.

Party Time

Whether you're going to a neighbor's dinner party or a holiday meal at your aunt's home, offer to bring an appetizer, salad, or side dish. Contributing a platter of chilled shrimp or a quinoa-vegetable salad will guarantee you at least one healthy choice. When I'm invited to a party, I always offer to bring a vegetable platter with homemade hummus or guacamole. The hostess is thrilled; it's one less thing for her to worry about. And I always take home an empty platter.

Drink Water

Water is an essential nutrient for good health. As I mentioned earlier, many people mistake hunger for thirst, and drinking a glass of water can often quell food cravings. Keep a bottle of water on your desk or in your car and drink from and refill it frequently. When traveling by air, take an empty water bottle and fill it from a fountain after you pass through security.

> *I learned that it is important and okay to put myself first. If I can't take care of myself, then I can't take care of my family. The adventure of trying new foods and recipes on the Healthy You program was awesome and inspired me to create some of my own— it's hard to mess up when using real foods! While weight loss is good, the awesome feeling of becoming and maintaining a healthy new version of myself makes me giddy. I've learned to drink water and lots of it. And now I'm always sure to have food prepped and ready to have as a snack or a meal.*
>
> KIM RYAN-PITEL

Eat Two Healthy Meals a Day

Before I developed the Healthy You Diet, weeklong vacations and business trips would set back my weight-loss efforts. These days I return without having gained an ounce. By following a few guidelines, I can keep my weight in check and still enjoy my vacation.

If possible, ask that the minibar and basket of snacks be removed from your hotel room and replaced with an empty refrigerator that you can fill with large bottles of water and healthy snacks.

Everyone wants to take a break from everyday routine while on vacation, especially when it comes to wining and dining. Though I take pleasure in eating and drinking while traveling, I make sure to eat healthy meals on most days. In the morning, I have oatmeal and fruit or some scrambled eggs. At lunch, I enjoy a big salad with grilled fish or sliced flank steak. This way, I can occasionally order something indulgent at dinner. If I allow myself to splurge at every meal, then I pack on the vacation pounds.

> *I was diagnosed with thyroid cancer 1 year ago. After surgery and treatments, I decided it was time to become healthy. I lost 80 pounds, but then I hit a plateau and just couldn't lose those last 30 pounds. I started the Healthy You Challenge and lost 19 pounds (9 pounds and 13 inches in the first 7 days!). I then continued on the program after the 2 weeks and lost 11 more pounds. I am so proud of my accomplishments.*
>
> JAIME HURST

Sleep

You may be surprised to learn that sleep plays an important role in weight loss and weight control. According to a 2011 study published in the journal *Obesity*, people who stay up late consume almost 250 more calories per day than those who go to bed early. That's an additional 91,250 calories a year, equivalent to 26 pounds!

Michael Breus, PhD, the clinical director of the sleep division at Arrowhead Health in Glendale, Arizona, says that lack of sleep causes your metabolism to function improperly. When you are sleep deprived, you also produce more of the hormone ghrelin and less of the hormone leptin. Ghrelin tells you when to eat, while leptin tells you when to stop, so being sleep deprived can actually make you want to eat more.

Research also shows that sleep is important for quality brain function. Think of your brain as a vacuum cleaner that needs to be emptied every night so it will work properly the next day. Other health benefits from a good night's sleep include improved memory, decreased stress, increased creativity, better athletic performance, and reduced anxiety and depression.

Train yourself to go to sleep at the same time every night and log a solid 7 to 8 hours. Avoid watching TV or reading on electronic devices; the glow from the light stimulates your brain and slows the release of the sleep-inducing hormone melatonin. Instead, read a printed book in low lighting or listen to quiet music. If you find a particular scent, such as lavender or grapefruit, soothing, then spray some in the air. Take a warm bath. Drink a cup of chamomile or other herbal tea. Having a regular evening routine and bedtime will help you get the sleep you need for health and weight loss.

Exercise

I developed the Healthy You Diet to work with or without exercise. Just the thought of physical activity keeps some people from trying to lose weight. While you can successfully lose weight without exercise, you'll reach your goal sooner if you combine some sort of fitness regimen with a healthy diet. A regular exercise program—going for a walk for 30 minutes 5 days a week or taking yoga or Pilates classes twice a week—will reduce stress, boost your energy levels, improve your mood, and help you get a solid night's sleep.

After I graduated from college and moved to New York, I gained so much weight that I no longer had the motivation to work out. No way was I going to put on spandex and be seen at the gym. One night, while chatting with my roommate, I learned that she, too, was desperately trying to lose weight. Once the cat was out of the bag, we made a pact to get up early 3 or 4 days a week and run together in Central Park. What had once been an easy jog for both of us when we were younger now left us exhausted and gasping for breath. We started by alternating walking and running for just 2 miles and then increased our distance bit by bit. After a few weeks, I noticed that I felt more energized during the day and slept better at night.

My roommate and I decided to sign up for a 5-K in Central Park. I can't remember how long it took me to run the race, but I do remember the feeling of exhilaration when I crossed the finish line. I've exercised regularly ever since. With my busy schedule, I try to be realistic and exercise 4 or 5 days a week. When I have the time, I might attend an hour-long exercise or yoga class or go for a bike ride or a long run. But more often than not, I go for a 30-minute run or fast walk. Working out is something I now look forward to rather than dread. Just 30 minutes of exercise makes a huge difference in my mood and my stress and energy levels, and it helps me maintain my weight.

If you're new to exercise or haven't worked out in ages, start slowly and build up gradually. Slip on a pair of comfy sneakers and take a walk—outdoors or on a treadmill. If you choose the treadmill, slowly increase the incline to get your heart rate up. Sign up for water aerobics at the Y. Take dance, Spin, or flexibility classes. To quiet your mind, try tai chi or meditation. There are hundreds of choices. Know that a combination of clean eating and regular exercise is the ultimate recipe for better health.

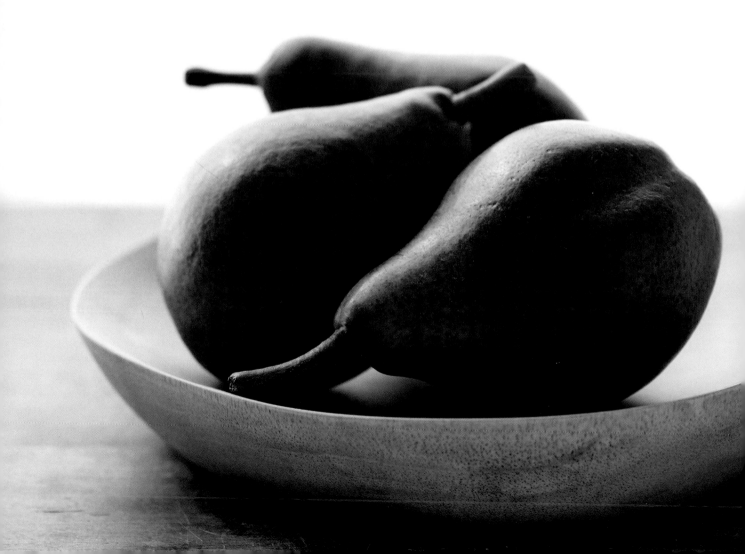

chapter

8

the healthy you pantry

One weekend morning, I came down to the kitchen to find my 5-year-old son frantically going through our pantry.

"What are you doing?" I asked.

He replied, "Daddy."

When I moved closer, I realized he was upset, so I asked, "What about Daddy?" He turned away from the pantry and looked up at me with his sad little face and teary eyes. He whimpered, "Daddy ate my potato chips!"

I did everything I could to suppress a smile, since potato chips aren't breakfast food at our house. "Luke," I said, "we will talk to Daddy and remind him not to eat your chips."

"Okay," he replied, "but why don't you get Daddy his own bag?" I decided it wasn't worth explaining that Daddy actually had his own bag of chips, but once it was empty, he went scavenging for more. I just couldn't bring myself to tell my son that his father was a potato chip addict.

I always say that when it comes to certain foods, "if it is around, it will be eaten." My husband never craves chocolate, cookies, cake, or other desserts, but if you step between him and a bag of Ruffles, you do so at your own peril. For him, chips are a trigger food. If there's a bag of potato chips in the pantry, he will eat them, even if it means stealing from a little boy.

Everyone I know has favorite foods that they love. Personally, I couldn't care less about potato chips, but if there's some chocolate or cookies in the pantry, I will find them and eat them. There's only one solution for avoiding temptation when it comes to your personal trigger foods: Don't keep them in the kitchen (or anywhere else in the house!).

To avoid temptation, remove temptation. Before you start the Healthy You Diet, give your pantry, refrigerator, and freezer a top-to-bottom "spring cleaning" and discard any foods that could sabotage your weight-loss goals. This approach has numerous benefits.

- When I remove trigger foods from my kitchen, I immediately feel better. Just knowing that there are no cookies to tempt me has a positive impact on my mental well-being.

- For those who find it difficult to remain focused on eating healthy foods when trying to lose weight, out of sight is out of mind. When life becomes overwhelming, do you usually reach for the ice cream in the freezer or the pretzels in the cupboard? If your trigger food isn't accessible, then you won't be able to eat it.

- You'll make space in your refrigerator and pantry for all the wholesome and nutritious foods that you'll be enjoying on the Healthy You Diet. The program is designed to introduce you to a variety of foods that you may be unfamiliar with. My hope is that once you embrace these new foods, you'll continue to enjoy them for the rest of your life.

Take 30 minutes to sort through the food in your kitchen. If you find items that will be eliminated—processed foods, diet beverages, and so on—during the Healthy You Diet, get rid of them now. I'm confident that a little pantry modification will leave you feeling good—and, more important, these adjustments are an essential step toward reaching your weight-loss goals.

You can reintroduce some of these foods after the 2 weeks and once you've learned to be more conscious about what you eat. Although my kids eat healthy meals most of the time, I allow them treats. There was a time when having cookies in the house would completely derail my healthy eating. But today I can keep them as special treats that the entire family can enjoy in moderation. This is something I could never have done before losing weight on the Healthy You Diet.

Buying Organic Fruits and Vegetables

I suggest buying organic produce, even though it's more costly. If you can't afford or choose not to buy all organic produce, try to buy organic for what the Environmental Working Group's Shopper's Guide to Pesticides calls the **Dirty Dozen.** According to the EWG, these 12 fruits and vegetables are known for their large amounts of pesticide residue.

Apples	Cucumbers	Potatoes
Bell peppers	Grapes	Snap peas (imported)
Celery	Nectarines (imported)	Spinach
Cherry tomatoes	Peaches	Strawberries

Try to buy organic versions of the Dirty Dozen. You'll significantly cut down on how much pesticide you ingest.

The EWG also lists 15 fruits and vegetables that contain the least amounts of pesticide residue. The **Clean Fifteen** are:

Asparagus	Corn	Onions
Avocados	Eggplant	Papayas
Cabbage	Grapefruit	Peas (frozen)
Cantaloupe	Kiwifruit	Pineapple
Cauliflower	Mangoes	Sweet potatoes

Many farmers use organic methods and grow pesticide-free fruits and vegetables but can't afford the fees—often many thousands of dollars—to have their farms certified organic by state and local governments. Talk to the growers at your local farmers' market and ask how many acres they work and how they grow their produce.

Healthy You Ingredients

Now that you've cleaned out your pantry and tossed all those highly processed foods, artificial sweeteners, and other unhealthy ingredients, it's time to stock up on clean, quality foods that will help you reach your weight-loss goals. Some of the ingredients—perhaps quinoa or avocado oil—on the Healthy You Diet may be new to you, but beans, brown rice, and unsweetened almond milk are just as important as fresh fruits and vegetables and lean proteins. All of them are available in supermarkets and health food stores. Here are some of my favorite ingredients that I keep stocked in my pantry.

Baking Powder, Gluten-Free

Gluten in baking powder? Where's the wheat? Baking powder is essentially composed of a dry acid and dry alkali (such as cream of tartar or bicarbonate of soda). When the baking powder in a batter or dough is moistened, the acid and alkali combust to create carbon dioxide, which helps the dough rise.

In addition to the active acid and alkali, an anticaking agent is included in the formula. Usually this ingredient is gluten-free cornstarch or potato starch, but it can also be a wheat starch, so check the label to be sure. The top three brands of baking powder (Rumford, Davis, and Clabber Girl) are all gluten free, so this isn't a prevalent problem but one that you should be aware of nonetheless.

Also, many brands use sodium aluminum sulfate as the dry alkali. If you have concerns about consuming aluminum, look for a brand that is aluminum free, too. Rumford contains neither aluminum nor gluten.

Beans

Beans are one of the healthiest foods, containing lots of protein, essential vitamins and minerals, and fiber. My pantry is always stocked with canned beans—cannellini, black beans, chickpeas. All I need is a can opener and a great meal is just minutes away.

Most canned foods contain high levels of sodium, and this is true of canned beans. Draining and rinsing the beans reduces the sodium by about one-third. Or you can buy low-sodium canned beans.

If you prefer taking the from-scratch route, you can cook dried beans. One pound of dried beans yields about 6 cups cooked. Store them (drained or with the cooking liquid) in $1\frac{1}{2}$-cup amounts, which is the equivalent of a 15-ounce can. Cooked beans can be refrigerated for up to 3 days or frozen for up to 3 months. (Thin lentils don't require soaking or precooking.)

To cook dried beans, start by giving them the once-over to check for unwanted stones or tiny dirt clods that may have slipped through during processing. I find the easiest way to do this is to spread the beans on a baking sheet, sort through them, and remove any foreign materials. Rinse the beans well under cold running water and drain.

Beans should be soaked before cooking, a step that makes them a bit easier to digest and helps them hold their shape. The old-fashioned way requires soaking the beans in a bowl of water for at least 4 hours or overnight, but the quick-soak method is much faster and just as good. Put the beans in a large saucepan and add enough cold water to cover by 2 inches to allow for expansion. Bring to a boil over high heat, then boil briskly for 2 minutes. Remove from the heat, tightly cover the pot, and let stand for 1 hour.

Return the drained beans to a large saucepan and add enough cold water to cover them by 2 inches. Bring to a boil over high heat. Reduce the heat to medium-low and partially cover the pot to keep the water from evaporating too quickly. Simmer the beans until tender, using the chart below. Keep in mind that the cooking time is always an estimate based on many factors, including the age of the beans, water hardness, and altitude. About 10 minutes before the beans are done, stir in 1 tablespoon of sea salt—unseasoned beans are very bland. Drain, reserving the cooking liquid if required by the recipe. Let the beans cool before storing.

Small beans (black, cranberry, great Northern, black-eyed peas)	45 min–1 hr
Medium beans (navy, pinto, small red)	1–1½ hr
Large beans (chickpea, red kidney, cannellini)	1½–2 hr

Brown Rice

Rice is one of the world's most consumed foods, but I wish that everyone ate brown rather than white rice! Most of the rice's nutrients reside in its brown skin, but with white rice, this is "polished" off during processing. In fact, most American brands of white rice are sprayed with vitamins B_1 and B_3 and iron to replace what was destroyed during milling and processing. That doesn't make any sense. There's really no excuse for buying white rice, since even basmati and jasmine are available in their natural brown states. Keep raw brown rice in a covered container in a cool, dry place for up to 2 to 3 months.

The many healthful properties of brown rice disappear when its skin is removed. Brown rice has been shown to be an antioxidant, which fights disease and slows aging. It has lots of fiber to fill you up and helps burn fat because it takes longer to digest and uses more energy to do so. The oils in brown rice help control cholesterol, which, in turn, keeps your heart in good operation. And it's an excellent source of manganese and selenium, essential dietary minerals that keep our bodies working well.

The length of its grain identifies the rice, which is also relative to its starch content. Long-grain rice has the least starch, so it cooks up into individual grains. Medium-grain rice has a moderate amount of starch, and its grains cling together. Short-grain rice, used for sushi and other dishes, is sticky and holds together when pressed. It's also called sweet or glutinous rice, even though it contains neither sugar nor gluten. These terms are used to differentiate it from standard "nonsticky" rice. I use sweet brown rice in my California rolls; regular long-grain brown rice won't hold together when pressed into shape. Any rice can be milled into flour. I use standard (not sweet) brown rice flour in my other recipes.

Since brown rice takes at least twice as long to cook as white rice (about 45 minutes, as opposed to 20), prepare more than you need for a single meal and store the leftovers. Transfer the cooked rice to zip-top plastic bags in convenient individual or family-size portions and refrigerate for up to 3 days or freeze for up to 3 months. Refrigerated or frozen rice can be easily reheated in a microwave for 3 minutes on high power.

For about twelve ½-cup servings of cooked brown rice, thoroughly rinse 2 cups rice in a wire sieve under cold running water. Transfer to a medium saucepan and add 5 cups water or vegetable broth and 1 teaspoon sea salt. (For six servings, use 1 cup rice, 2½ cups liquid, and 1 teaspoon sea salt.) Bring to a boil over high heat. Tightly cover the pan and reduce the heat to low. Simmer for about 45 minutes, or until the liquid is absorbed and the rice is tender. Remove from the heat and let stand, covered, for 5 minutes. If any liquid remains, drain the rice in the sieve. Fluff the rice with a fork and serve or place in storage containers.

Brown Rice Pasta

Just because you are on a wheat-free diet doesn't mean you can't enjoy pasta. There are many whole grain pastas made without wheat—brown rice, quinoa, corn, and potato—in a number of shapes and sizes, including spaghetti, fettuccine, fusilli, penne, elbows, and shells. Brown rice pasta is my favorite.

Read the package label to be sure that the pasta wasn't prepared in a facility that processes wheat, barley, or rye, especially if you're trying to eliminate gluten. All three contain gluten, and you could inadvertently ingest traces of these grains. Brown rice pasta is a whole grain pasta, so you get all of the benefits that come with it, including a healthy dose of dietary fiber. Whenever you think you don't have anything in the house for dinner, brown rice pasta, cooked and mixed with vegetables and fresh herbs, can come to the rescue.

Regardless of its many benefits, all pasta has calories, so measure carefully before cooking. Two ounces or ¾ cup of uncooked brown rice pasta contains about 200 calories. I find that every brand requires a different cooking time, so follow the package directions, taking care not to overcook.

Chipotles in Adobo

The amount of hot and smoky flavor packed into a small can of chipotles in adobo is amazing. Chipotles are red-ripe jalapeño peppers that have been smoked over an oak fire. While they are sold in this dried state or ground into a powder, most often they are canned with adobo, a vinegary and spicy sauce. Among the spiciest chiles around, chipotles are used sparingly.

When chopping chipotles, take care not to touch them, or wear rubber gloves to protect your hands. After handling chipotles, never touch sensitive parts of your body, especially your eyes. Using the tip of your chopping knife, spear a chipotle and transfer it and any clinging adobo to a chopping board. Chop the chipotle, seeds and all. Scrape up the chopped chili with the sharp edge of the knife and add to the food as required. Leftover chiles can be stored with the adobo in a small covered container and refrigerated for a few weeks or frozen for up to 3 months.

Coconut Flour

Ground from dehydrated coconut flesh with the fat removed, this high-fiber flour is also low in carbohydrates. The fiber can soak up a lot of liquid, so keep that in mind when cooking with it. After opening the bag, refrigerate or freeze coconut flour in an airtight container.

Coconut Palm Sugar

Made in Southeast Asian countries from the boiled and dried sap of the coconut palm tree, this is a coarsely granulated brown sugar with a light caramel flavor. It comes from a different tree than Thai or Vietnamese palm sugar, which is usually sold in chunks and must be grated before using. Unlike white cane sugar, coconut palm sugar is very minimally processed. You'll find it at Asian markets and many natural food stores.

Although most of the recipes on the Healthy You Diet are sugar-free, I do use coconut palm sugar in some of the wheat- and dairy-free desserts for a healthy indulgence.

Coconut Water

Often confused with coconut milk, coconut water is the clear, refreshing liquid you hear sloshing inside young, green coconuts. Naturally sweet and fat free, coconut water is easy for the body to digest. With 60 calories per 11-ounce serving, it shouldn't be gulped indiscriminately. Leftover coconut water should be refrigerated in a covered container for up to 4 days.

Flax Meal

This highly nutritious food is just ground flaxseed. While you can buy whole flaxseed and grind it as needed in a coffee mill, flax meal is much more convenient. To avoid spoilage, store it in the refrigerator or freezer, where it will keep for a few months.

Honey

Honey gets its main flavor from the bees' nectar source—wildflower honey tastes different from buckeye, for example. Some honey is very strongly flavored, and you will get the most reliable results with a blended honey, which is made from different varieties.

Honey keeps indefinitely covered and at room temperature. If it crystallizes, just place the container in a bowl of very hot water, changing the water occasionally if needed, until the crystals melt and the honey is smooth again. Because some honey containers may not be made to withstand high temperatures, do not attempt to microwave crystallized honey without first transferring it to a microwave-safe bowl.

Milk Substitutes

Whether you're lactose intolerant, have a milk allergy, or just want to cut back on your consumption of dairy, today you can choose from more milk alternatives then ever before. Some of the most popular include almond, soy, and rice milk. Additionally, oat and hemp milk are becoming more mainstream.

Almond milk: This dairy-free beverage is made from ground almonds that have been steeped in water to extract their flavor and then strained. The nutty flavor is mild; the consistency, thin and creamy. Unsweetened plain almond milk is the most versatile; choose it over sweetened or flavored ones.

Soy milk: Made from soybeans, soy milk can be substituted for cow's milk. The jury is still out, however, as to whether soy milk and other soy foods are healthy additions to our diets. Of the thousands of studies done on soy foods, some show that eating soy has no harmful effects, while others indicate that genetically modified soybeans (most of the world's crop) are dangerous. When I became pregnant with my daughter, my doctor asked that I cut back on my consumption of soy, which is how I came to love almond milk. Speak to your health care provider about the pros and cons of consuming soy.

Rice milk: This milk substitute is usually made from brown rice. Its thin consistency makes rice milk great as an oatmeal topping but not ideal for baking or cooking.

Coconut milk: A staple in Asian and Indian cuisines, coconut milk is prepared from freshly grated coconut squeezed to a rich, thick liquid. It's sold in cans in the supermarket's Asian aisle. Be sure to shake the can well, because the thick coconut fat rises to the top and should be incorporated with the thinner milk below before using. Transfer opened coconut milk to a covered container and refrigerate for up to a week. Coconut milk is high in calories, so use a low-fat version. Don't confuse coconut milk with cream of coconut, a very sweet and gooey concoction used mainly in tropical drinks.

Hemp milk: Hemp is a good source of omega-3 and omega-6 fatty acids, as well as calcium. Although almond, soy, rice, and coconut milk can be found in large grocery stores, you may have to go to a health food store to locate hemp milk.

Oat milk: This milk substitute is gaining in popularity. It is high in fiber and is lactose free, but those who are gluten intolerant should avoid it.

Nuts and Nut Butters

In many cases, what a cook calls a nut (almonds, walnuts, and peanuts included) a botanist would call a drupe or legume. To simplify, let's just say that a nut has a hard shell surrounding an edible seed. Nuts are an important part of a wheat-free lifestyle because of the flavor and bulk they provide, but they are also high in fat and calories, so enjoy them with a bit of restraint.

Shelled nuts are, of course, the easiest to use. For the longest storage, pack them in a resealable plastic bag and refrigerate for up to 6 months (or freeze for up to a year).

When purchasing nut butters, look for all-natural brands that have not been hydrogenated. These are easy to spot, because the oil is visible in a thin layer at the top of the jar. This oil can make a mess when you try to stir it back into the butter. Get in the habit of storing nut butter upside down, so the oil ends up at the bottom, which makes it much easier to stir and incorporate. Or transfer the entire contents of the jar to a medium bowl with deep sides, whisk everything together with a handheld stick blender, and then scrape the combined nut butter back into its jar. Do not refrigerate nut butter, as it gets hard and impossible to mix.

Oils

Some plants can be processed to remove their naturally occurring oils, and these fats can be used for cooking. Each oil has a slightly different flavor and purpose, so I keep several types on hand. Remember that we do need some fat in our diets—the trick is to concentrate on the heart-friendly, monounsaturated oils.

Heat and light can rapidly age oils, so store these products in a cool, dark place, where they'll usually keep for about 3 months. In fact, some manufacturers even pack their oils in colored glass bottles to diminish exposure to strong light. Oil can be refrigerated for longer storage, but it can turn cloudy and semisolid until it is brought back to room temperature. You can tell rancid oil by its unappetizing aroma and flavor. It can't be saved, so just toss it and buy a new bottle.

Avocado oil: This oil, processed from avocado flesh, has a buttery flavor that makes it a good choice for sautéing, and it also makes delicious salad dressing.

Coconut oil: Although coconut oil is a saturated fat, it is from a plant source and much better for you than animal saturated fats such as butter or lard. Pure (that is, unrefined, sometimes called virgin) coconut oil, made from coconut palm flesh, has become the oil of choice for many cooks. It can be used for sautéing and in baked goods, but it doesn't have a strong coconut flavor. As a saturated fat, it is solid at cool room temperature but will liquefy above 76°F, and this low melting point is one reason it is the base of so many cosmetics that will be spread on the skin. Coconut oil contains antioxidants to give it a shelf life of about 2 years at room temperature; don't refrigerate it or it may be too hard to use easily.

To melt coconut oil, simply place the covered container in a bowl of hot tap water, weigh it down with a plate so it is half submerged, and let it stand for a few minutes. The coconut oil around the edges will melt fairly quickly, and you can pour off the amount needed.

Olive oil, extra-virgin: Olives are grown throughout the Mediterranean (in Italy,

Spain, France, Portugal, Greece, and Turkey) and in the warmest areas of California, so there are many different brands that depend on the variety of the olive and where it is grown. It is difficult to recommend a single kind of olive oil because the "best" one is usually a matter of personal taste. Extra-virgin olive oil has been minimally refined and is basically olives pressed without any heat or chemicals to extract the oil. You can tell this oil by its green color—regular (formerly called pure) olive oil is golden and has been more highly refined.

Peanut oil: Another oil with a high smoke point, peanut oil has a very mild, nutty taste. Look for cold-pressed peanut oil, which indicates that it has been minimally processed. Most supermarket brands are highly refined.

Quinoa

This tiny, protein-packed seed is often sold in its common white variety, but you'll also find red, black, and rainbow, as well as a combination of all three. It cooks up into fluffy, tender grains and can be added to salads and soups or served as an accompaniment to seafood, poultry, or meat. Quinoa provides all of the essential eight amino acids (most plants have only seven, missing lysine), making it especially useful in health-conscious, plant-based cooking. All quinoa must be rinsed to remove its natural coating of a very bitter chemical compound called saponin. Do this even if the packaging states "prerinsed." Put the raw quinoa in a fine-mesh sieve and rinse it well under cold running water, stirring with your fingers to be sure that all of the grains come in contact with the water. Drain well before cooking.

For four servings of about ½ cup each, rinse and drain ¾ cup quinoa. Combine the quinoa, 2 cups water or vegetable broth, and a large pinch of salt in a saucepan. Bring to a boil, then reduce the heat to low. Cover and cook for 15 to 20 minutes, or until the quinoa has absorbed the liquid and is tender. Remove from the heat and let stand, covered, for 5 minutes. Fluff with a fork and serve.

Quinoa is so versatile. For breakfast, top a serving with a poached or fried egg. Substitute quinoa for other grains in salad recipes. Top with any cooked vegetables and some grilled chicken, lean steak, or seafood.

Quinoa Flour

Made from milled quinoa seeds, quinoa flour is often mixed with other flours to replace wheat when baking. For example, the dough for Mediterranean Flatbread Pizzas (page 192) uses a combination of quinoa and brown rice flours. Store quinoa flour in the refrigerator after opening, but bring it to room temperature before using.

Quinoa Pasta

Quinoa flour can be combined with other gluten-free flours to make excellent, high-protein pasta. One brand sells a wide variety of shapes, so a hankering for, say, rotelle, can be satisfied. Quinoa pasta has a firm texture similar to the traditional version, so it can stand up to heavier sauces. Just follow the package directions for cooking.

Sea Salt

While vacationing on the stunning Caribbean island of Bonaire, I took my kids to see the 200-foot-tall mountains of sea salt drying in the sun. At first they didn't believe that the huge white piles against the bright blue sky were salt, until it was explained to them that sea salt is harvested from evaporated seawater.

I specify sea salt in my recipes because it isn't processed like table or kosher salts, which have additives such as anticaking agents. Sea salt is sometimes labeled with its country of origin. Some types have more trace minerals, and choosing, say, French sea salt over British is a matter of personal preference.

When buying sea salt, be sure to get the fine crystals, as the coarse ones need to be ground. Use a grinder if you prefer, but there is no culinary reason to do this, because minerals (like salt and unlike herbs and spices) contain no essential oils or aromas that are released during grinding.

Soy Sauce versus Tamari

The basic description of tamari is that it is a wheat-free and gluten-free version of soy sauce, but that's not always accurate.

Soy sauce is specifically fermented for bottling from a mash of soybeans, wheat, water, and yeast. There are some gluten-free brands available. Tamari is a by-product of miso, a fermented soybean paste that is a salty seasoning in Japanese cuisine. As the paste ferments in a huge vat, liquid tamari forms and is removed. While wheat is usually not used in miso production, some producers do include it in their mash, so double-check the label to ensure that the tamari does not include wheat or gluten.

There are flavor differences between soy sauce and tamari, too. Because of its longer fermentation period, tamari has a smoother, more complex taste. If you've ever found soy sauce to be too salty and harsh, then you will probably prefer tamari for its flavor, as well as the fact that it is gluten free.

Toasting Nuts and Seeds

It takes only a few minutes to toast nuts and seeds. This easy procedure adds lots of flavor to your food. Thin seeds can be toasted in a skillet, but heftier nuts are more efficiently toasted in an oven.

To toast nuts such as walnuts, hazelnuts, and blanched almonds, spread on a rimmed baking sheet. Bake in a preheated 350°F oven, stirring occasionally, for 10 to 15 minutes, or until the nuts smell toasty and are lightly browned. (For a small amount of nuts—say, ½ cup or so—you can use a toaster oven, spreading the nuts on the oven's small tray.)

To toast seeds such as sesame and pumpkin, preheat a skillet over medium heat. Add the seeds and stir occasionally for 2 to 3 minutes, or until the seeds are fragrant and lightly browned. Immediately transfer to a plate to cool completely before using. Do not let them cool in the skillet or they may burn from the residual heat.

Vinegars

Having a wide range of vinegars in your pantry is one of the easiest ways to add variety to your cooking. Good cooks know that a bit of acidity just makes food taste better. (Think of that squeeze of lemon on your grilled fish and you'll know what I mean.) Here are the vinegars that I use most often.

Apple cider vinegar: Traditionally made from cider that is allowed to sour, apple cider vinegar doesn't have a lot of fruit flavor. It's useful as an all-purpose vinegar for salads and seasoning vegetables such as cooked greens. If you wish, purchase an unfiltered type, which contains a harmless, cloudy film called the mother, a by-product of the natural fermentation.

Balsamic vinegar: This popular vinegar has an irresistible sweet-sour flavor. It is made in small batches from the sweet trebbiano grape, then aged for many years in wood barrels and allowed to evaporate into a thick syrup. You'll know authentic balsamic by its label (it will say *tradizionale*) and its price tag. Supermarket balsamic is flavored red wine vinegar, but it works well for dressings and cooking. In between the tradizionale and supermarket varieties is aged balsamic, which you will find at specialty grocers and online. This balsamic is aged for 8 years, and while not cheap, it has a lot of the same flavor characteristics as the very expensive tradizionale and is worth the extra few bucks.

Rice vinegar: Fermented from a rice-based liquid, this is one of the mildest vinegars, with about 4.5 percent acidity (compared with 6 percent for wine vinegar). While there are Chinese rice vinegars, it is the Japanese version that you will find at the supermarket. Pale yellow, it gives food a gentle tang. Look carefully at the label to be sure that you are getting unseasoned or plain rice vinegar. Avoid seasoned rice vinegar, which is flavored with salt and sugar and specifically used to make sushi rice.

White wine/champagne vinegar: Both of these have a mild acidity and rounded flavor, making them more useful than the typical red wine vinegar, which can be harsh (especially the inexpensive ones). Although white and champagne vinegars look similar, there are subtle differences. White wine vinegar is made from Chardonnay grapes and is slightly stronger in flavor. "Clear" champagne vinegar is actually made from red wine grapes—the juice doesn't color because the dark skins are strained out after crushing. I keep both on hand.

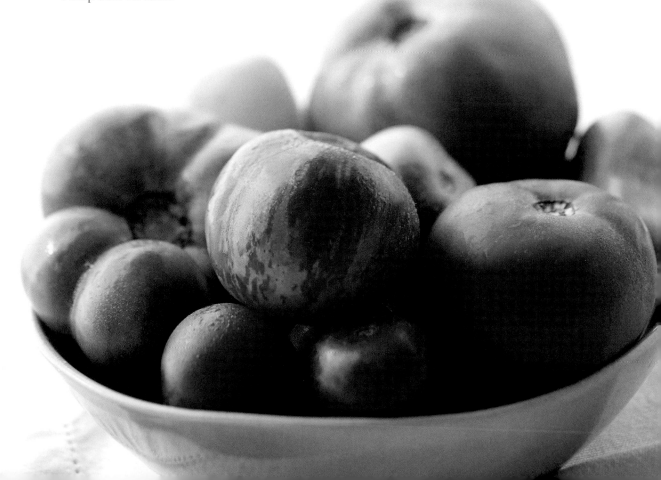

the clean life

Living the clean life is about fueling your body so you can become the best and healthiest you possible. The 14-day Healthy You Diet is how you get started. But it's not just a 14-day diet. It's a better way to a slimmer, healthier, more energetic you.

That's why this is more than a diet book. It's a cookbook that you'll actually want to use—with clean, healthy, amazing-tasting recipes!

Many of these recipes have become staples in my family's diet. I have a feeling that they will appear frequently on your table, too. They're nutrient dense, so you can feel good about serving them to friends and family.

Most important, my Healthy You Diet recipes are geared toward your good health, building a better relationship with food, never feeling deprived, and giving you a new appreciation for how good the right food can make you look and feel.

Ideally, the diet should be followed as written. Life, however, doesn't always allow for that. It's okay to make some modifications that better fit your life's schedule. However you follow it, my program will help you take the first step in your journey toward clean eating, weight loss, and a more satisfying life.

The following section includes more than 100 of my favorite recipes, including those in the 14-day program. From Banana-Maple-Pecan Pancakes (page 82) to Wild Rice–

Spinach Soup (page 104) to Grilled Salmon and Citrus Salad (page 151) and Roasted Vegetable Pasta (page 188), you will find dishes to serve and enjoy at any occasion, from a backyard barbecue (Chicken Skewers with Honey-Lime-Chile Sauce, page 171) to a cocktail party (Scallop Ceviche, page 207, or Cherry Tomato Bruschetta, page 203) to a kid's birthday party (Triple Chocolate Brownies, page 224).

I know what it's like to be unhealthy and overweight—I've shared those stories with you—but I also know what it's like to feel truly well and vibrant. My hope is that through the Healthy You Diet and with these recipes, you, too, will feel at your best.

Pick and choose from any of these recipes once you've completed the first 14 days. You will be amazed at what a difference clean eating can make!

The following key will help you decide what recipes are right for you.

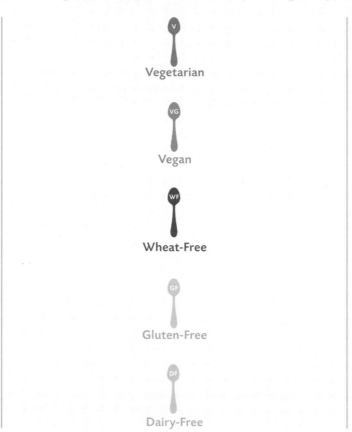

Vegetarian

Vegan

Wheat-Free

Gluten-Free

Dairy-Free

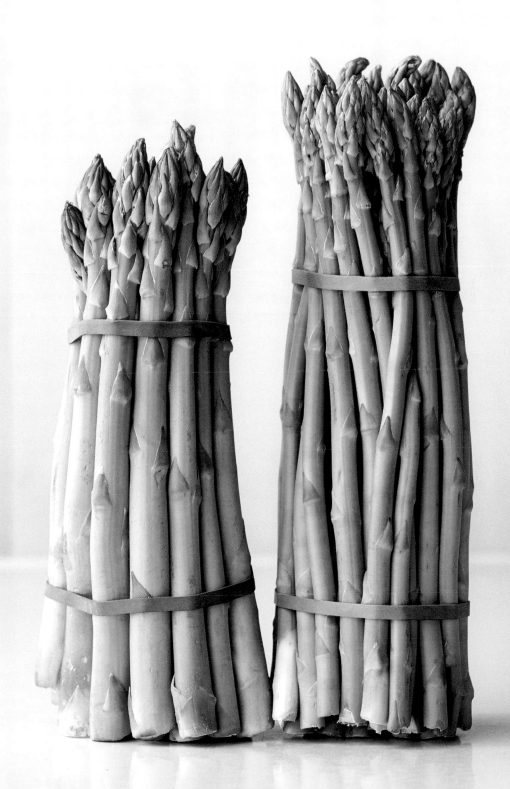

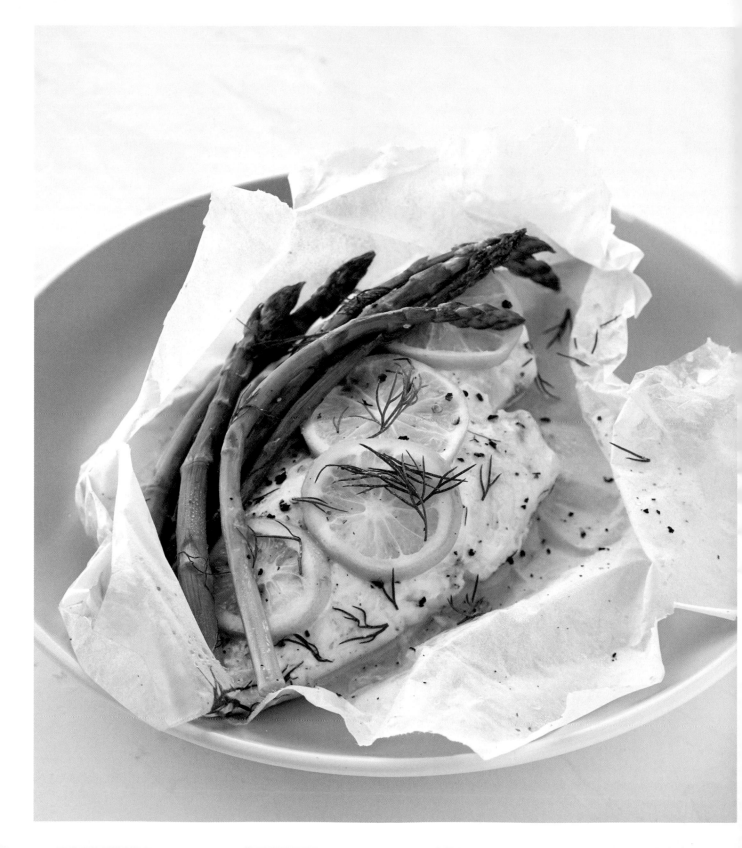

part two

the healthy you recipes

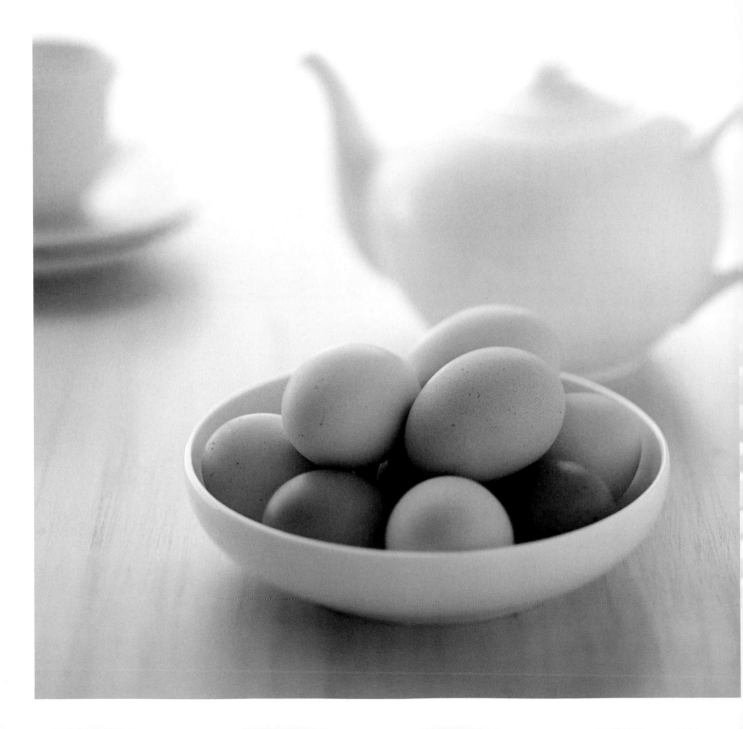

morning meals

I've always been a huge proponent of eating breakfast. Now that I have young children, I've become even more pro-breakfast. It's important to send my kids off to school with the energy they need to start the day and remain focused and productive. The following dishes will start your day off with oomph! The Banana-Maple-Pecan Pancakes (page 82) have a special place in my heart: My 5-year-old son helped me develop the recipe, and now he always makes them on the weekends.

Cranberry-Orange Granola

Making your own granola means you can avoid store-bought brands that contain sugar, wheat products, and preservatives. Many brands of rolled oats are made in mills that also process wheat products, meaning that the oats may be contaminated with wheat. Be sure to buy gluten-free oats. Also purchase juice-sweetened dried cranberries rather than those with added sugar. Here's where reading those food labels makes a huge difference!

TOTAL TIME: 40 MINUTES

1¾ cups gluten-free rolled oats

¾ cup chopped walnuts

½ cup chopped pecans

½ cup raw pumpkin seeds

½ cup unsweetened flaked coconut

2 tablespoons chia seeds

½ cup all-fruit orange marmalade

2 tablespoons coconut oil

1½ teaspoons ground cinnamon

1¼ teaspoons ground ginger

¼ teaspoon sea salt (optional)

½ cup juice-sweetened dried cranberries

Preheat the oven to 325°F. Line a 15" × 10" baking pan with parchment paper.

In a large bowl, combine the oats, walnuts, pecans, pumpkin seeds, coconut, and chia seeds. Mix well.

In a small saucepan, combine the marmalade, oil, cinnamon, ginger, and salt (if desired). Heat over low heat, stirring constantly, until the oil and marmalade melt. Pour over the oat mixture, stirring well to coat.

Spread the granola in the pan as evenly as possible. Bake, stirring once, for 25 to 30 minutes, or until lightly browned.

Remove the pan from the oven and gently stir in the cranberries. Let the granola cool completely on the pan. Store in an airtight container.

Makes 12 servings (about 4 cups)

Grain-Free Granola

Once baked, this crunchy granola of sunflower and chia seeds, walnuts, almond flour, and dried blueberries is broken up into sweet tidbits. Enjoy it with unsweetened almond milk in the morning. Because it's almost like candy, kids love this as an after-school snack.

TOTAL TIME: 45 MINUTES

¾ **cup coarsely mashed bananas (1–2 bananas)**

¼ **cup brown rice syrup**

2 **teaspoons ground cinnamon**

1 **cup raw sunflower seeds**

1 **cup walnut pieces**

¾ **cup almond flour**

3 **tablespoons chia seeds**

½ **cup juice-sweetened dried blueberries**

Preheat the oven to 350°F. Line a 15" × 10" baking pan with parchment paper.

In a blender or food processor, combine the bananas, rice syrup, and cinnamon. Blend or process until smooth.

In a large bowl, whisk together the sunflower seeds, walnuts, almond flour, chia seeds, and blueberries. Add the banana mixture and stir to coat the seeds and nuts.

With moistened hands, spread the mixture in the pan into a rectangle approximately 12" × 9". Bake for 30 minutes, or until the bottom is lightly browned.

Remove from the oven and turn off the oven. Using a pancake turner, turn the granola over and break into large pieces. Return the granola to the still-hot oven for 10 minutes to continue baking in the residual heat.

Cool the granola in the pan set on a rack. Break into clusters and refrigerate in an airtight container. The granola becomes crisper as it cools.

Makes 10 servings (about 5 cups)

BREAKFAST
DAYS
2, 4 & 11

Oatmeal with Fresh Berries and Almond Milk

I prefer the chewy texture of steel-cut oats, also called Irish oats, but when time is short in the morning, I often use instant oatmeal. With some berries and milk, a bowl of oatmeal satisfies me until lunchtime. Steel-cut oats can be made the night before if you wish.

TOTAL TIME: 15 TO 25 MINUTES

1½ cups water

½ cup gluten-free steel-cut oats

½ cup mixed berries

½ cup unsweetened almond milk

In a saucepan over medium-high heat, bring the water to a boil. Add the oats, cover, and reduce the heat to low. Cook, stirring occasionally, for 10 to 20 minutes. The length of time needed to cook the oats depends on the type of oats and how chewy you like them. Steel-cut oats take longer than rolled oats.

Remove the covered pan from the heat and let it sit for a few minutes. Serve the hot oatmeal topped with the berries and milk.

Makes 1 serving

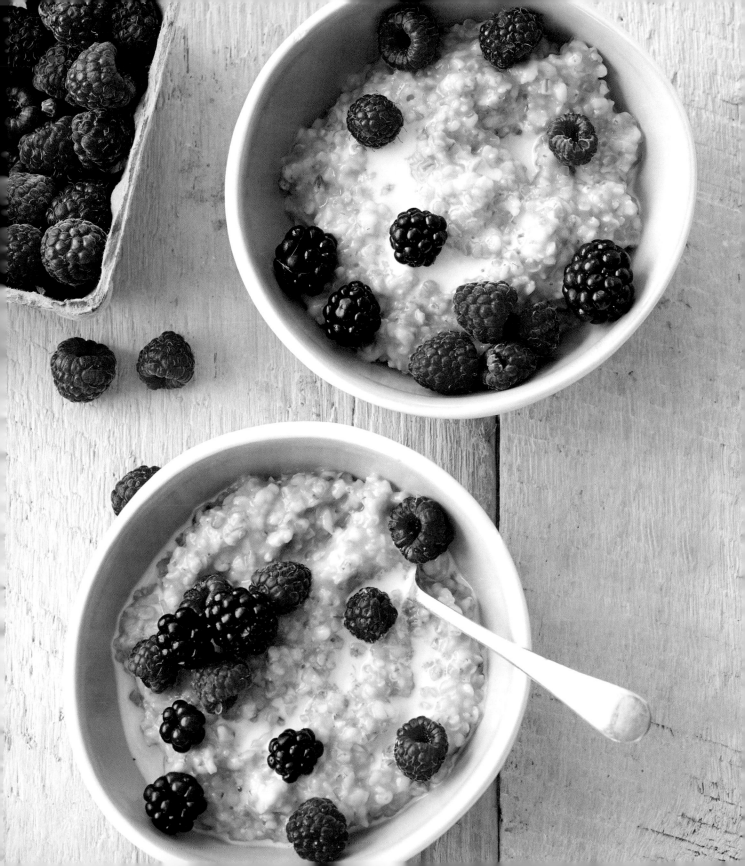

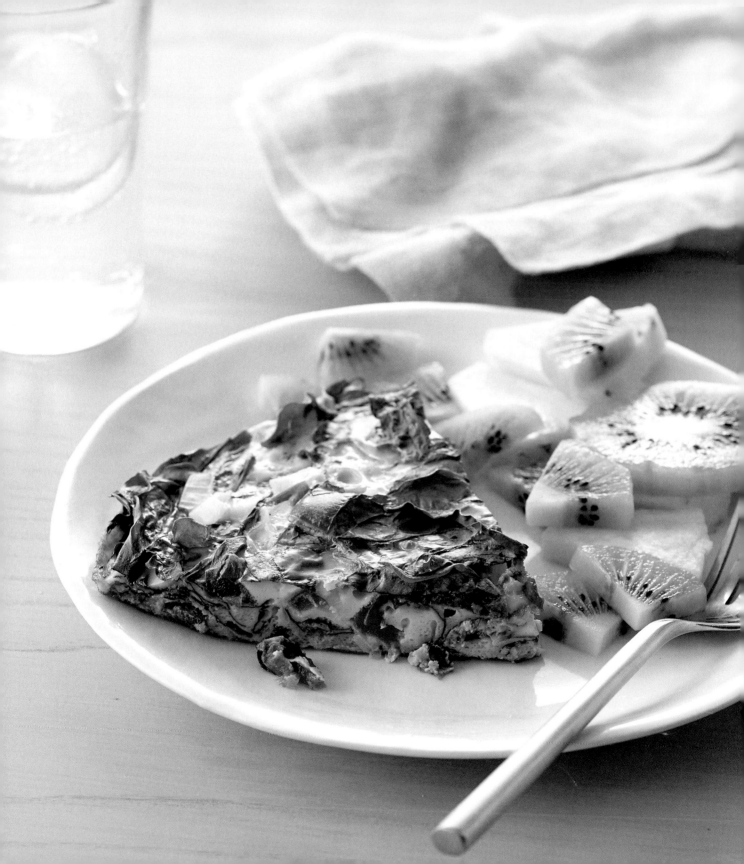

Spinach, Tomato, and Basil Frittata

In a frittata, an Italian open-face omelet, all of the vegetables and herbs are whisked together with the eggs, and then the mixture is poured into a skillet. The frittata's bottom is cooked on the stovetop, and then the skillet is put into the oven so the eggs brown and puff.

TOTAL TIME: 15 MINUTES

6 large eggs

2 large egg whites

4 ounces fresh baby spinach leaves, stems removed

2 tomatoes, chopped

½ cup finely chopped onion

1 tablespoon chopped fresh basil leaves

¼ teaspoon sea salt

¼ teaspoon ground black pepper

½ teaspoon extra-virgin olive oil

Preheat the oven to 400°F.

In a mixing bowl, whisk together the eggs and egg whites. Fold in the spinach, tomatoes, and onion. Stir in the basil, salt, and pepper.

Coat a large ovenproof, nonstick skillet with the oil and heat the skillet over medium heat. Pour the egg mixture into the skillet and cook for 1 minute, or until the eggs start to set. Transfer the skillet to the oven and bake for 5 to 6 minutes, or until the top is golden and puffy.

Remove the frittata from the oven and let it stand for 5 minutes before cutting into wedges and serving.

Makes 4 servings

Vegetable Omelet

Although tomato, onion, and bell pepper are the suggested fillings below, feel free to use any leftover vegetables—broccoli, cauliflower, mushrooms, zucchini—and herbs.

TOTAL TIME: 10 MINUTES

2 large eggs

1 large egg white

1 teaspoon extra-virgin olive oil, divided

1 small tomato, chopped

2 tablespoons chopped onion

2 tablespoons chopped red or yellow bell pepper

8–10 baby spinach leaves

Pinch of sea salt

In a small bowl, whisk the eggs with the egg white and set aside.

Coat a small nonstick skillet with ½ teaspoon of the oil and heat over medium heat. Cook the tomato, onion, and pepper for 4 to 5 minutes, or until tender. Transfer to a bowl.

Wipe the skillet and then coat it with the remaining ½ teaspoon oil. Set over medium-high heat. Add the reserved eggs and cook for 2 minutes, lifting the edges of the omelet as it sets and allowing the uncooked egg to flow to the edges of the skillet.

As the center of the omelet begins to set, spoon the cooked vegetables on one side of the omelet and top with the spinach. Season with the salt. Gently fold 1 side of the omelet over the other. Cook for 1 minute to let the omelet set. Slide the omelet from the skillet to a plate and serve.

Makes 1 serving

Vegetable Scramble

Unlike an omelet or a frittata, this quick scramble uses vegetables that are cooked first, and then the eggs are poured on top and gently cooked. This is another great way to use up leftover vegetables in a morning meal.

TOTAL TIME: 10 MINUTES

2 large eggs

Pinch of sea salt

Pinch of ground black pepper

1 teaspoon extra-virgin olive oil

¼ cup chopped onion

½ cup baby spinach

½ cup chopped tomatoes

In a bowl, whisk together the eggs, salt, and pepper and set aside.

Coat a small nonstick skillet with the oil and heat over medium heat. Cook the onion, stirring frequently, for 2 to 3 minutes, or until translucent. Add the spinach and tomatoes and cook for 2 minutes, or until the spinach is wilted. Pour the reserved eggs over the vegetables. Gently stir and cook the eggs and vegetables for 1 to 3 minutes, or until desired doneness.

Makes 1 serving

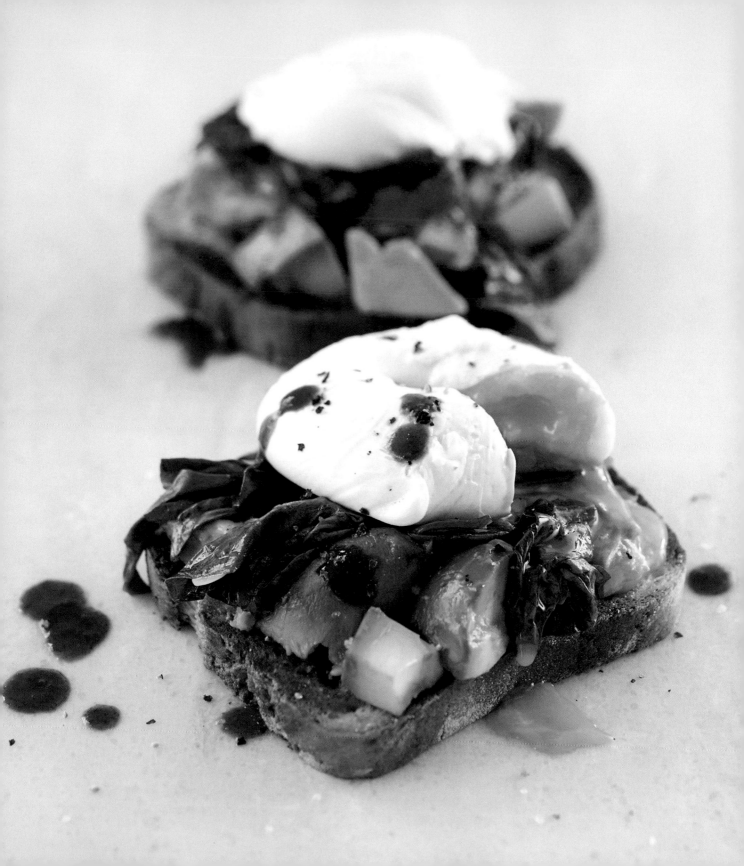

Poached Egg, Avocado, and Spinach Toasts

I like to make poached eggs on the weekends when there's a bit more time for a leisurely breakfast or lunch. Poached eggs and spinach on toast are a traditional combination, but I add some avocado for another texture.

TOTAL TIME: 15 TO 20 MINUTES

1 ripe avocado, peeled, pitted, and cubed

Juice of ½ lemon

¼ teaspoon sea salt + more to taste

1 tablespoon extra-virgin olive oil

3 cloves garlic, thinly sliced

¾ pound spinach, stemmed and rinsed, but not dried

Ground black pepper to taste

2 tablespoons white vinegar

4 large eggs

4 slices gluten-free bread, toasted

Hot sauce (optional)

In a small bowl, combine the avocado with the lemon juice and ¼ teaspoon salt. Set aside.

In a large skillet over medium heat, heat the oil. Add the garlic and cook for 1 minute, or until fragrant. Add the spinach and cook until just wilted, using tongs to turn the spinach. Transfer to a bowl and season with salt and pepper to taste. Wipe the skillet clean.

To poach the eggs, fill the clean skillet halfway with water and add the vinegar. Bring to a boil over high heat. Break the eggs into 4 small bowls. Remove the pan from the heat and gently slide the eggs into the skillet. Cover the pan tightly and let the eggs sit for 4 minutes, or until the whites are set and the yolks are still runny.

Spread the reserved avocado on the toast. Spoon the warm spinach mixture on top. Using a slotted spoon, carefully transfer the eggs from the skillet to the toast. Serve with the hot sauce (if desired).

Makes 4 servings

Banana-Maple-Pecan Pancakes

Since my 5-year-old son is a connoisseur of pancakes, I wasn't sure what he would think of this dairy-, gluten-, and wheat-free recipe. The first time I made them he devoured them, and now he asks me to make them every weekend. When shopping, note that products labeled "flax meal" and "flaxseed meal" are the same item and can be used interchangeably.

TOTAL TIME: 15 TO 20 MINUTES

½ cup mashed ripe bananas (1–2 bananas)

2 large eggs

½ cup almond butter

¼ cup flax meal

1 tablespoon pure maple syrup, plus more for serving

1½ teaspoons gluten-free baking powder

1 teaspoon ground cinnamon

½ teaspoon vegetable oil

¼ cup chopped pecans

Sliced bananas, for garnish

In a food processor, combine the bananas, eggs, almond butter, flax meal, maple syrup, baking powder, and cinnamon. Process until smooth.

Heat a griddle or skillet over medium-high heat and brush with the oil. Using a ¼-cup measure, ladle the pancake batter onto the griddle. Cook for 6 minutes, turning once, or until golden brown.

Serve the pancakes with maple syrup and top with the pecans and banana slices.

Makes 2 servings

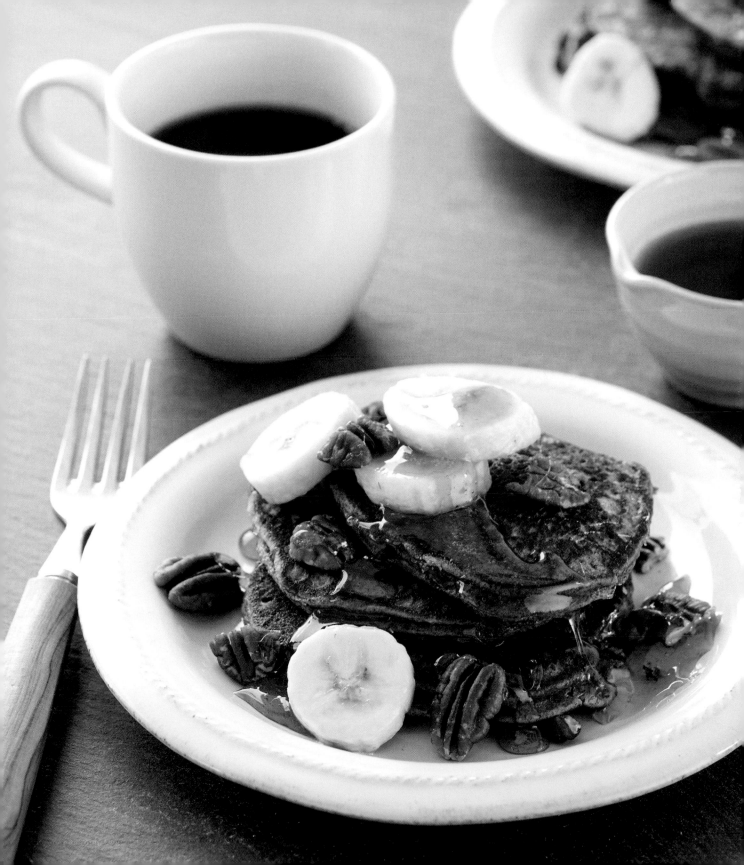

Blueberry-Lemon-Almond Pancakes

Pancakes made with almond flour, which is finely ground almonds, are lighter than those made with wheat flour. Personalize them by substituting raspberries for the blueberries and orange extract for the lemon. These are a great weekend treat for the entire family.

TOTAL TIME: 15 TO 20 MINUTES

½ cup unsweetened almond milk

1 large egg

2 teaspoons honey

½ teaspoon lemon extract

⅔ cup almond flour

5 tablespoons flax meal

1 teaspoon gluten-free baking powder

⅛ teaspoon sea salt

⅓ cup + ¼ cup blueberries

1 teaspoon vegetable oil

2 tablespoons maple syrup

In a small bowl, whisk together the almond milk, egg, honey, and lemon extract.

In a large bowl, mix together the almond flour, flax meal, baking powder, and salt. Stir the milk mixture into the flour mixture. Do not overmix. Let the batter rest for 5 minutes. Gently fold in ⅓ cup of the blueberries.

In a large skillet or griddle over medium heat, heat the oil. Ladle the batter into the skillet using a ¼-cup measure. Cook for 6 minutes, turning once, or until golden brown. Reduce the heat if the pancakes are cooking too quickly. Drizzle with the maple syrup and garnish with the remaining ¼ cup blueberries.

Makes 2 servings

Apple-Oat Bread

Apples and nuts taste great together, and in this easy-to-make bread, the pairing is outstanding. Oat flour and almond flour give the bread a light texture and even better flavor. A slice of this bread is perfect for breakfast or a snack.

TOTAL TIME: 1½ HOURS

1 cup gluten-free oat flour

1 cup almond flour

½ cup coconut palm sugar

2½ teaspoons apple pie spice

1 teaspoon gluten-free baking powder

½ teaspoon baking soda

½ teaspoon sea salt

3 large eggs

1½ cups unpeeled, shredded apple (about 1 large or 2 small apples)

¾ cup chopped walnuts, divided

3 tablespoons melted coconut oil

Preheat the oven to 350°F. Line the bottom and short ends of an 8" × 4" loaf pan with parchment paper.

In a medium bowl, whisk together the oat flour, almond flour, sugar, spice, baking powder, baking soda, and salt.

In a large bowl, whisk the eggs. Add the apple, ½ cup of the walnuts, and the oil. Mix well. Add the dry ingredients to the egg mixture and stir gently to combine. Pour the batter into the pan and smooth the top. Scatter the remaining ¼ cup walnuts over the top of the loaf. Bake for 45 to 55 minutes, or until a wooden pick inserted in the center of the loaf comes out clean. Let the bread cool in the pan set on a rack for 10 minutes. Remove the loaf from the pan and cool completely on the rack before slicing.

Makes 12 servings

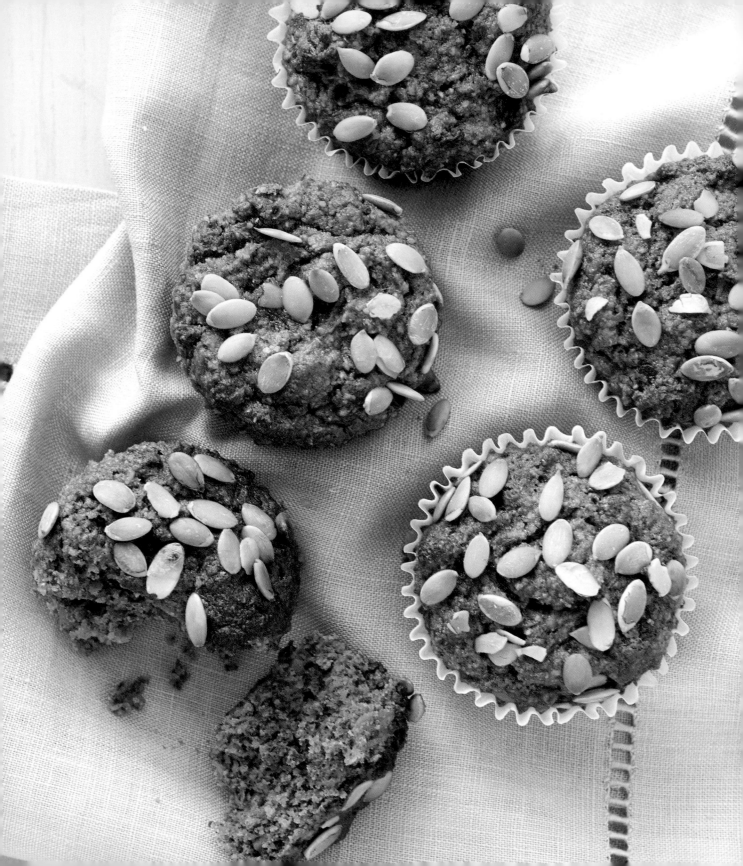

Sweet Potato Muffins

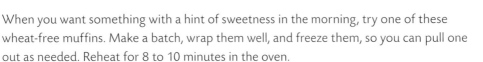

When you want something with a hint of sweetness in the morning, try one of these wheat-free muffins. Make a batch, wrap them well, and freeze them, so you can pull one out as needed. Reheat for 8 to 10 minutes in the oven.

TOTAL TIME: 45 MINUTES

1¾ cups almond flour

¾ cup flax meal

⅔ cup coconut palm sugar

2 teaspoons gluten-free baking powder

2 teaspoons pumpkin pie spice

1 teaspoon ground cinnamon

½ teaspoon sea salt

½ cup golden raisins

1½ cups shredded sweet potato

3 large eggs

¼ cup melted coconut oil

¼ cup fresh orange juice

¼ cup raw pumpkin seeds

Preheat the oven to 350°F. Place paper liners in a 12-cup muffin pan.

In a large bowl, whisk together the almond flour, flax meal, sugar, baking powder, pumpkin pie spice, cinnamon, and salt. Stir in the raisins.

In a medium bowl, stir together the sweet potato, eggs, oil, and orange juice. Add to the flour mixture, stirring well to combine. Do not overmix.

Divide the batter evenly among the paper liners, filling them about three-quarters full. Sprinkle the pumpkin seeds on the tops of the muffins. Bake for 30 minutes, or until a wooden pick inserted in the center of a muffin comes out clean. Cool in the pan set on a rack for 5 minutes. Remove the muffins from the pan and let them cool completely on the rack.

Makes 12 muffins

Blueberry-Banana Muffins

Who doesn't love blueberry muffins? And who doesn't love banana muffins? Put the two fruits together and bite into a muffin that says "good morning," both healthfully and deliciously.

TOTAL TIME: 45 MINUTES

3 cups almond flour

½ cup coconut palm sugar

2½ teaspoons gluten-free baking powder

1 teaspoon ground cinnamon

¼ teaspoon sea salt

1 cup mashed ripe bananas (2 bananas)

3 large eggs

2 tablespoons melted coconut oil

1 cup fresh blueberries

Preheat the oven to 325°F. Place paper liners in a 12-cup muffin pan.

In a medium bowl, whisk together the flour, sugar, baking powder, cinnamon, and salt.

In a large bowl, combine the bananas, eggs, and oil. Stir until well mixed. Add the dry ingredients to the banana mixture and stir gently to combine. Fold in the blueberries but do not overmix.

Divide the batter evenly among the paper liners, filling them about three-quarters full. Bake for 25 to 35 minutes, or until a wooden pick inserted in the center of a muffin comes out clean. Cool in the pan set on a rack for 5 minutes. Remove the muffins from the pan and let them cool completely on the rack.

Makes 12 muffins

chapter

smoothies and juices

Although I love traditional breakfast foods like eggs, oatmeal, and muffins, I've discovered that a nutrient-dense smoothie or juice gives me plenty of energy to start the day, but without the heaviness I sometimes feel with a bigger breakfast. Plus, both smoothies and juices can be a great midafternoon snack—the perfect cure for the late afternoon lull. These rich, creamy smoothies and refreshing, vibrant juices take very little time to prepare but are immensely satisfying.

Magic Mango Smoothie

This refreshing smoothie is just the pick-me-up needed in midafternoon.

TOTAL TIME: 5 MINUTES

½ cup unsweetened almond milk

2 tablespoons fresh orange juice

½ cup fresh or frozen cubed mango

½ frozen banana

4–6 ice cubes

In a blender, combine the almond milk, orange juice, mango, banana, and ice cubes. Blend until smooth. Pour into a tall glass.

Makes 1 serving

Pineapple-Avocado Smoothie

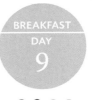

Pineapple and avocado are a unique combination, but once you try this smoothie, you'll love its bright, rich flavor.

TOTAL TIME: 5 MINUTES

½ avocado, peeled and pitted

½ banana

¼ cup fresh or frozen pineapple cubes

½ cup water

4–6 ice cubes

In a blender, combine the avocado, banana, pineapple, water, and ice cubes. Blend until smooth. Pour into a glass and enjoy.

Makes 1 serving

Comfort Smoothie

This rich, creamy, and dairy-free smoothie tastes more like a banana-nut muffin. Enjoy it without guilt, but with pleasure.

TOTAL TIME: 5 MINUTES

1 cup unsweetened almond milk

1 frozen banana

2 teaspoons flax meal

1 teaspoon vanilla extract

1 teaspoon ground cinnamon

1 teaspoon honey

2–4 ice cubes

In a blender, combine the almond milk, banana, flax meal, vanilla, cinnamon, honey, and ice cubes. Blend until smooth. Pour into a glass and enjoy.

Makes 1 serving

Peanut Butter–Chocolate Smoothie

VG WF GF DF

When I was a kid, my dad would always let my sister and me get a chocolate-covered frozen banana rolled in peanuts whenever we were at an amusement park. This protein-packed power shake brings back those great memories.

TOTAL TIME: 5 MINUTES

1 **cup unsweetened almond milk**

1 **scoop dairy-free chocolate protein powder**

1 **tablespoon natural peanut butter**

1 **frozen banana**

4–6 **ice cubes**

In a blender, combine the almond milk, protein powder, peanut butter, banana, and ice cubes. Blend until smooth. Pour into a tall glass.

Makes 1 serving

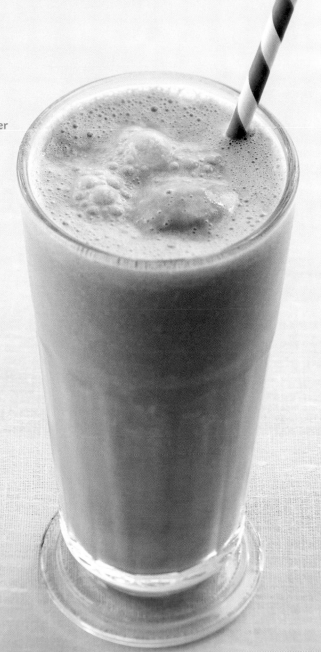

Kiwi-Melon Smoothie

Icy and refreshing, this drink falls somewhere between a smoothie and a juice. It's perfect for a warm day. My kids love the slushy texture.

TOTAL TIME: 5 MINUTES

1 **cup unsweetened coconut water**

1 **kiwifruit, peeled**

½ **cup cubed honeydew melon**

4–6 **ice cubes**

In a blender, combine the coconut water, kiwi, honeydew, and ice cubes. Blend until smooth. Pour into a tall glass.

Makes 1 serving

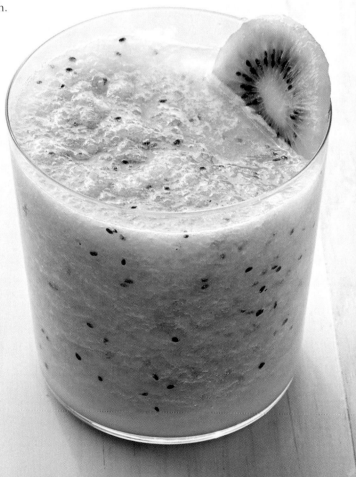

Strawberry-Banana Smoothie

The strawberry-banana combination is one of the most popular smoothie blends. This one has some orange juice for a bright touch.

TOTAL TIME: 5 MINUTES

4–5 fresh or frozen strawberries

½ banana

½ cup unsweetened almond milk

2 tablespoons fresh orange juice

4 ice cubes

In a blender, combine the strawberries, banana, almond milk, orange juice, and ice cubes. Blend until smooth. Pour into a glass and enjoy.

Makes 1 serving

Very Berry Smoothie

Smoothies full of berries rank among everyone's favorites. This one is no exception.

TOTAL TIME: 5 MINUTES

3–4 fresh or frozen strawberries

¼ **cup fresh or frozen blueberries or raspberries**

½ **banana**

½ **cup unsweetened almond milk**

4 **ice cubes**

In a blender, combine the strawberries,
blueberries or raspberries, banana,
almond milk, and ice cubes.
Blend until smooth.
Pour into a glass and enjoy.

Makes 1 serving

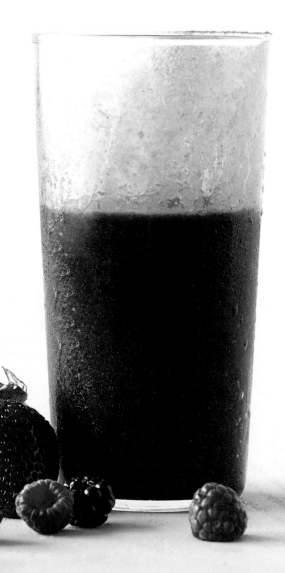

Super Green Juice

Green juices are hugely popular these days, and with good reason. They are bursting with direct-from-the-source goodness from vegetables and fruit. This one, made with kale and a green apple, tastes as fresh and green as it sounds.

TOTAL TIME: 5 MINUTES

4 large kale leaves

1 green apple, quartered and cored

1 rib celery

½ cucumber

½ lemon

In a juicer, juice the kale, apple, celery, cucumber, and lemon. Serve in a tall glass. If you enjoy your juice cold, pour it over ice.

Makes 1 serving

Radiant Red Juice

A mix of fruits and vegetables gives this juice just the right combination of sweet and savory.

TOTAL TIME: 5 MINUTES

1 cup fresh or frozen mixed berries, such as blueberries, raspberries, and blackberries

1 green apple, quartered and cored

1 rib celery

½ cucumber

½ lemon

1 cup baby spinach leaves

In a juicer, juice the berries, apple, celery, cucumber, lemon, and spinach. Serve in a tall glass. If you enjoy your juice cold, pour it over ice.

Makes 1 serving

ABC: Apple, Beet, and Celery Juice

Apples and celery are juicing staples. When you add a beet to the mix, this juice comes alive in color and flavor. It provides plenty of potassium, vitamin C, and fiber.

TOTAL TIME: 5 MINUTES

3 large kale leaves

2 ribs celery

1 beet (including leaves), halved

1 apple, quartered and cored

¼ lemon

In a juicer, juice the kale, celery, beet, apple, and lemon. Serve in a tall glass. If you enjoy your juice cold, pour it over ice.

Makes 1 serving

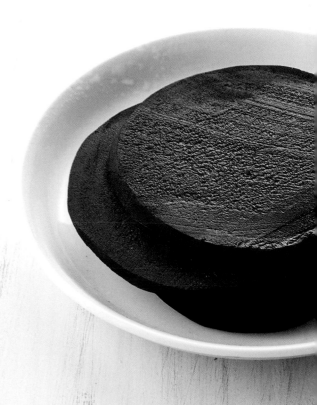

Easy Being Green Juice

Cucumber, green apple, and chard are the greens in this healthy juice. Carrots are included for another layer of sweetness.

TOTAL TIME: 5 MINUTES

2 large carrots

1 green apple, quartered and cored

1 small cucumber

4 Swiss chard leaves

¼ lemon

In a juicer, juice the carrots, apple, cucumber, chard, and lemon. Serve in a tall glass. If you enjoy your juice cold, pour it over ice.

Makes 1 serving

chapter

soups, sandwiches, and wraps

A bowl of soup is a satisfying one-dish meal, especially when it's made with plenty of vegetables, beans, or grains. On the Healthy You Diet, bread is used for a sandwich only on Day 1. After that, gluten-free bread wraps, rice paper, nori, and vegetable leaves are substituted for bread in sandwiches. My personal favorites are Tortilla Soup (page 108) and Shrimp Summer Rolls with Almond Dipping Sauce (page 124).

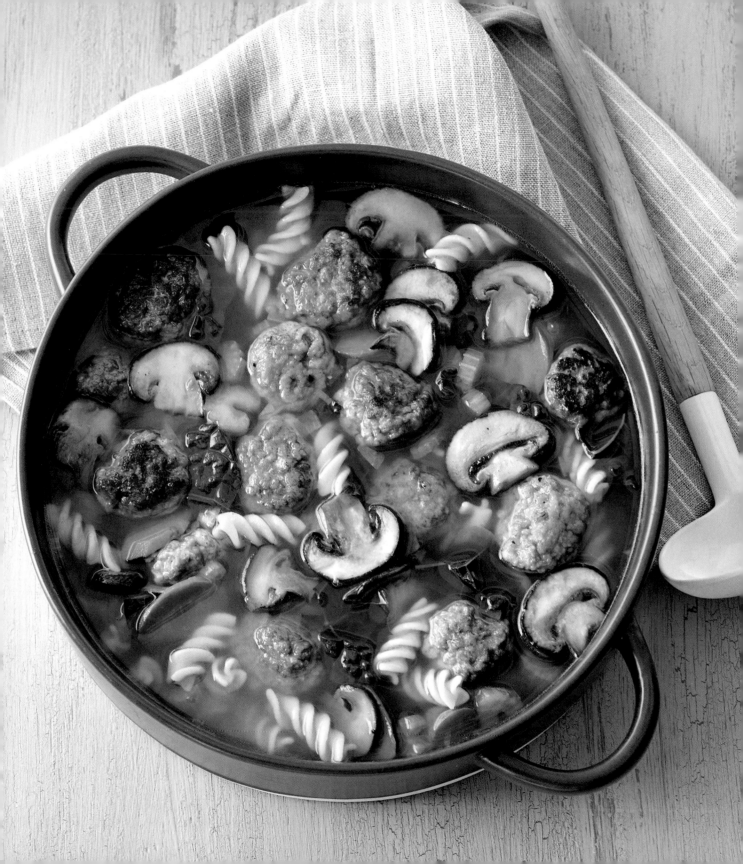

Chicken Meatball–Noodle Soup

Chicken noodle soup is always comforting and warming, but small chicken meatballs make this version satisfying for lunch or a light dinner.

TOTAL TIME: 1 HOUR

1 pound ground chicken	6 cups low-sodium chicken broth
Ground white pepper	½ cup sliced mushrooms
Sea salt	½ cup thinly sliced celery
1 tablespoon extra-virgin olive oil	2 kale leaves, thinly sliced
1 yellow onion, chopped	8 ounces brown rice pasta, such as rotini, small elbows, or broken spaghetti
1 cup thinly sliced carrots	

In a medium bowl, combine the chicken with ¼ teaspoon pepper and salt to taste. Shape into 12 small balls.

In a Dutch oven over medium-high heat, heat the oil. Cook the meatballs, turning occasionally, until browned. Transfer to a plate and set aside. Add the onion and cook, stirring frequently, for 4 to 5 minutes, or until translucent. Add the carrots and cook, stirring frequently, for 1 minute. Add the broth, mushrooms, celery, and kale. Season to taste with salt and pepper. Bring to a boil, reduce the heat, and simmer for 15 minutes, or until the vegetables are tender.

Meanwhile, prepare the pasta according to package directions. Drain, cover, and set aside.

Gently add the reserved meatballs to the soup and simmer for 10 to 12 minutes, or until they are cooked through. Add the reserved pasta to the soup, stir to mix, and heat through before ladling into 4 soup bowls.

Makes 4 servings

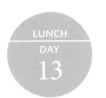

Wild Rice–Spinach Soup

Nothing warms the heart (and body) like comforting soup. This one requires some advance preparation, so plan ahead. Soaking the wild rice helps reduce its cooking time by about half. If you choose to skip this step, cook the wild rice as directed on the package. Soaking the walnuts—the longer, the better—gives the soup a creamy texture. Both steps are worth it.

TOTAL TIME: 50 MINUTES + SOAKING TIME

¾ cup uncooked wild rice

½ cup walnut pieces

1 tablespoon extra-virgin olive oil

2 carrots, chopped

2 ribs celery, thinly sliced

½ pound cremini or button mushrooms, sliced

1 yellow onion, chopped

2 cloves garlic, minced

4 cups low-sodium vegetable broth

1 bay leaf

1 teaspoon dried thyme

½ teaspoon sea salt

¼ teaspoon ground black pepper

¼ teaspoon red-pepper flakes

3 cups fresh spinach leaves

Grated peel of 1 small lemon

In a large bowl, cover the wild rice with enough water to cover by 2" and let it soak for at least 6 hours or overnight. Drain and rinse. Set aside.

In another bowl, cover the walnuts with enough water to cover by 1". Cover the bowl and set aside at room temperature to soak for at least 1 hour or up to 12 hours. Drain the walnuts and rinse well. Transfer the walnuts to a blender and puree until very smooth, about 2 minutes. Set aside.

In a large saucepan over medium heat, heat the oil. Cook the carrots, celery, mushrooms, and onion for 6 minutes, or until softened. Stir in the garlic and cook for 1 minute. Add the broth, bay leaf, thyme, salt, black pepper, red-pepper flakes, and reserved rice. Bring to a rapid simmer, reduce the heat, cover, and simmer for 30 minutes, or until the rice is tender. Remove and discard the bay leaf. Stir in the reserved walnuts, spinach, and lemon peel. Cook for 3 to 4 minutes, or until the spinach is wilted and the soup is heated through.

Makes 6 servings

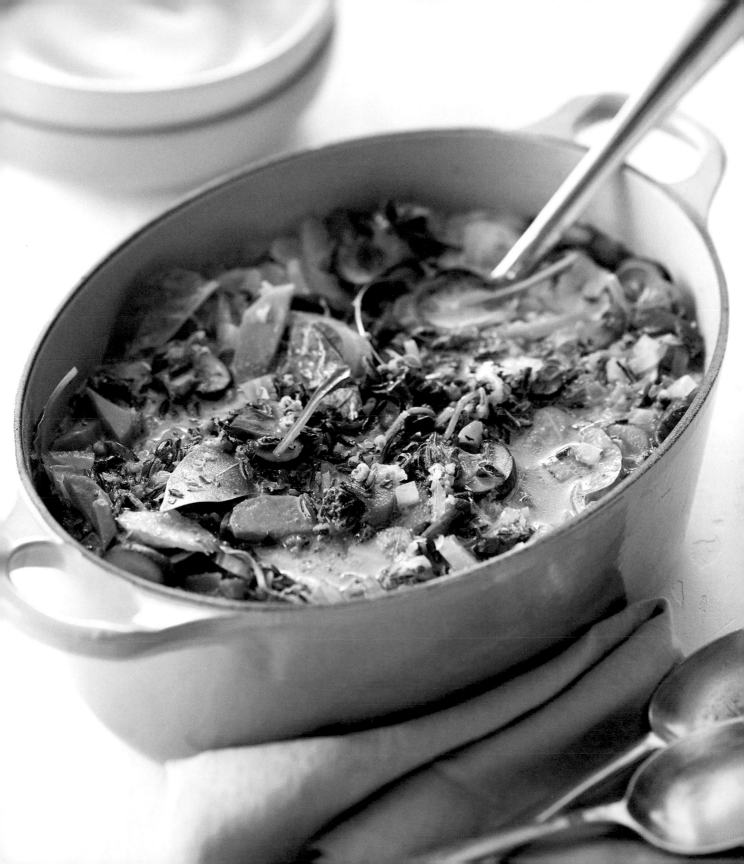

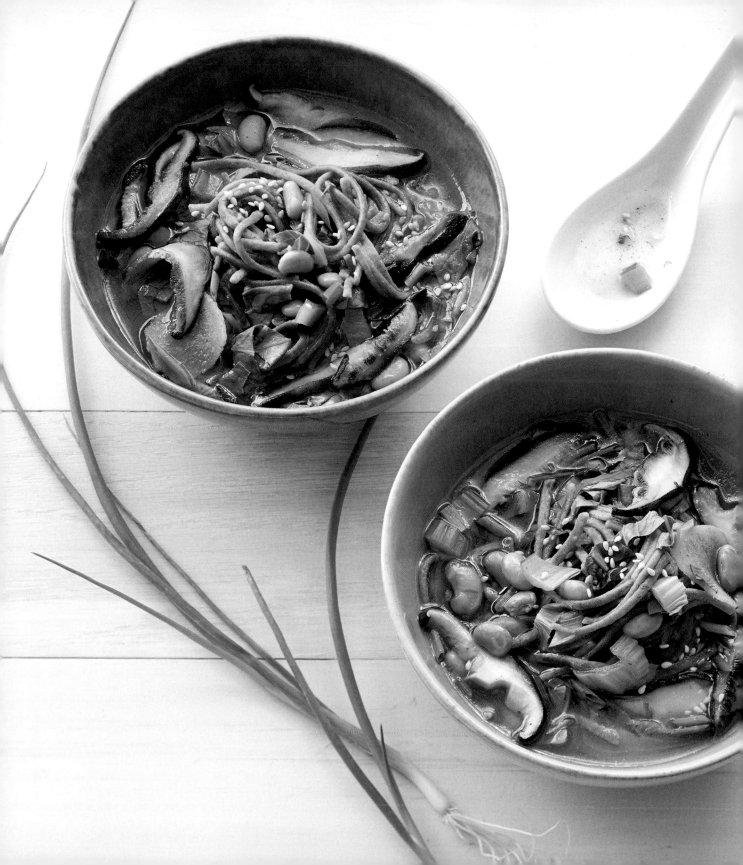

Shiitake Mushroom and Soba Noodle Soup

Soba is the Japanese name for buckwheat. Buckwheat is technically a seed, not a grain, which makes it gluten-free. Buckwheat comes from an entirely different botanical family than wheat. Make sure that the soba noodles you purchase are 100 percent buckwheat; some varieties may contain wheat. Miso, a Japanese soybean paste that comes in all sorts of colors and depth of flavors, will keep in the refrigerator for 6 months once opened.

TOTAL TIME: 30 MINUTES

6 ounces 100% buckwheat soba noodles

1 cup shelled frozen edamame

2 teaspoons peanut oil

3 baby bok choy, stems and leaves separated and sliced

½ pound shiitake mushrooms, stemmed and sliced

2 cloves garlic, minced

1" fresh ginger, thinly sliced

1 teaspoon Chinese five-spice powder

¼ teaspoon red-pepper flakes

6 cups water

3 tablespoons white or yellow miso

2 scallions, thinly sliced

2 teaspoons toasted sesame oil

1 tablespoon sesame seeds

In a large saucepan, prepare the soba noodles according to package directions. Drain in a colander and immediately rinse with cold water. Set aside.

In a small saucepan, cook the edamame according to package directions. Drain in a colander and set aside.

Return the large saucepan to the stovetop and heat the peanut oil over medium heat. Cook the bok choy stems, mushrooms, garlic, and ginger, stirring constantly, for 3 minutes. Add the spice powder and red-pepper flakes and stir for 30 seconds. Add the water and the bok choy leaves and bring to a gentle simmer.

Put the miso in a small bowl. Remove 1 cup of the hot water from the saucepan and whisk with the miso until smooth. Add to the saucepan and stir. Add the scallions, sesame oil, reserved soba noodles, and reserved edamame and stir to combine.

Ladle the soup into 4 soup bowls and garnish each with a sprinkle of sesame seeds.

Makes 4 servings

Tortilla Soup

Whenever I stayed at the Hyatt Hotel in Scottsdale, Arizona, I always ordered the tortilla soup. I found myself craving it once I returned home, so I developed this healthy wheat-free, dairy-free, vegan version.

TOTAL TIME: 45 MINUTES

1 tablespoon extra-virgin olive oil

1 white onion, chopped

2 cloves garlic, chopped

2 carrots, chopped

1 poblano chile pepper or red bell pepper, chopped (wear plastic gloves when handling)

2 jalapeño chile peppers, seeded and finely chopped (wear plastic gloves when handling)

1 teaspoon ground cumin

½ teaspoon sea salt

¼ teaspoon ground black pepper

2 cups frozen corn kernels or fresh corn kernels from 2–3 ears

2½ cups canned (rinsed and drained) or cooked pinto beans (page 54)

1 can (28 ounces) diced tomatoes

3 cups low-sodium vegetable broth

1 teaspoon dried oregano

4 corn tortillas, cut into ½" strips

1 avocado, pitted, peeled, and cubed

⅓ cup chopped cilantro

1 lime, sliced into 6 wedges (optional)

In a large saucepan over medium heat, heat the oil. Cook the onion for 6 minutes, or until softened and golden. Add the garlic, carrots, poblano or bell pepper, and jalapeño peppers and cook for 1 minute. Stir in the cumin, salt, and black pepper and cook for 30 seconds. Add the corn, beans, tomatoes, broth, and oregano. Bring to a boil, reduce the heat to medium low, and simmer for 20 minutes, or until the vegetables are tender.

Meanwhile, preheat the oven to 400°F. Arrange the tortilla strips on a baking sheet. Bake for 2 minutes, or until crisp.

Divide the soup among 6 soup bowls. Top with the avocado, cilantro, and tortilla strips. Serve with lime wedges (if using).

Makes 6 servings

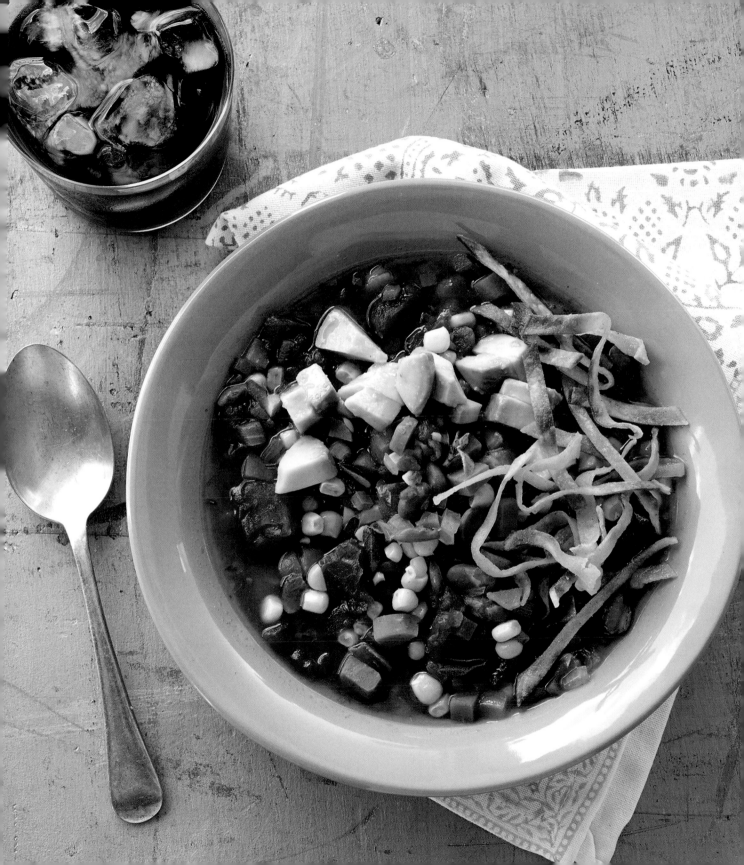

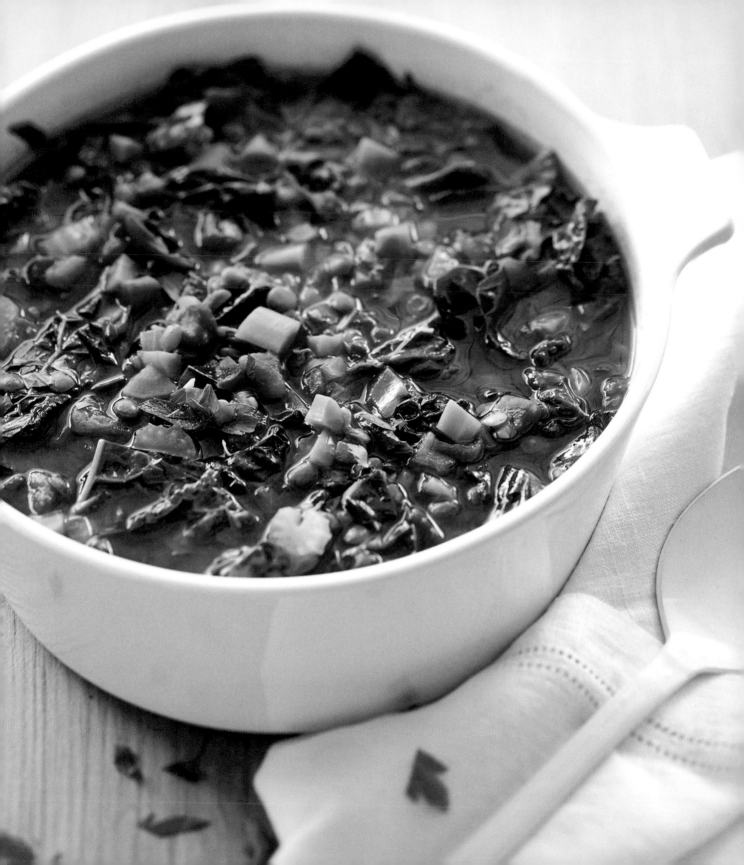

Lentil and Kale Soup

Lentils have the third highest level of protein of any legume or nut. Lentils come in a wide variety of colors, and they offer a great vegetarian option. Pair them with kale and some aromatic vegetables, and you have yourself a super-nutritious meal. The white wine gives the soup a hint of acidic flavor. If you choose to omit it, increase the vegetable broth to 6 cups.

TOTAL TIME: 50 MINUTES

1 tablespoon extra-virgin olive oil

1 large yellow onion, chopped

2 carrots, chopped

2 ribs celery, sliced

2 cloves garlic, minced

1 cup dry white wine (optional)

5 cups low-sodium vegetable broth

1 cup lentils, rinsed and picked over

1 can (14.5 ounces) diced fire-roasted tomatoes

1 bay leaf

1 teaspoon dried thyme

½ teaspoon sea salt

½ teaspoon ground black pepper

¼ teaspoon red-pepper flakes (optional)

4 large kale leaves, ribs removed and torn into 2" pieces

2 teaspoons balsamic vinegar

⅓ cup roughly chopped flat-leaf parsley

In a large saucepan over medium heat, heat the oil. Cook the onion, carrots, and celery, stirring frequently, for 6 minutes, or until softened. Add the garlic and cook for 1 minute.

Pour in the wine (if desired), increase the heat to medium high, and boil for 5 minutes, or until the wine has reduced by half.

Add the broth, lentils, tomatoes, bay leaf, thyme, salt, black pepper, and red-pepper flakes (if desired). Bring the soup to a boil, reduce the heat to medium low, cover, and simmer for 30 minutes, or until the lentils are tender but not mushy.

Remove and discard the bay leaf. Stir in the kale and balsamic vinegar. Cook until the kale has wilted. Divide the soup among 6 soup bowls and garnish with the parsley.

Makes 6 servings

Chicken Curry Soup

Fish sauce, *nuoc nam* in Vietnamese and *nam pla* in Thai, imparts an extra layer of flavor to this warming soup. An essential condiment in Southeast Asian food, it's available in super-markets and Asian grocery stores everywhere. This soup only gets better after a day or two in the refrigerator. It's tasty on the day it's made, of course, but if you are looking for something to make ahead, here's the ticket.

TOTAL TIME: 40 MINUTES

1 tablespoon peanut oil

1 pound boneless, skinless chicken thighs, cut into 1" pieces

1 red onion, chopped

½ pound small red-skinned potatoes, quartered

2 carrots, sliced diagonally into 2" pieces

1 large red bell pepper, seeded and thinly sliced

2 cloves garlic, minced

1 tablespoon finely chopped fresh ginger

1½ tablespoons curry powder

½ teaspoon sea salt

¼ teaspoon ground cinnamon

¼ teaspoon ground red pepper

¼ teaspoon ground black pepper

4 cups low-sodium chicken broth

1 can (13.5 ounces) coconut milk

1 tablespoon fish sauce (optional)

Juice of ½ lime

⅓ cup loosely packed, sliced fresh basil leaves

In a large saucepan over medium heat, heat the oil. Cook the chicken for 5 minutes, or until no longer pink. Remove the chicken from the pan and set aside.

Add the onion to the pan and cook, stirring, for 6 minutes, or until softened. Add the potatoes, carrots, bell pepper, garlic, and ginger and cook, stirring, for 1 minute. Stir in the curry pow-der, salt, cinnamon, red pepper, and black pepper and cook for 30 seconds. Add the broth, increase the heat to medium high, and bring to a boil. Reduce the heat to medium low, cover, and simmer for 20 minutes, or until the potatoes are tender.

Add the coconut milk, fish sauce (if desired), and reserved chicken and cook for 5 minutes, or until hot. Stir in the lime juice and basil before serving.

Makes 6 servings

Vegetable Soup

I have to thank my sister Michele for this easy vegetable soup. As a busy working mother, she is always looking for healthful meals her kids will like. They love this soup, and who wouldn't, bursting as it is with fresh vegetables? Michele usually makes it with carrots, green beans, and tomatoes—vegetables her kids love—but you can substitute your favorites or those you have on hand. Perhaps the best thing about this soup is that it tastes even better the second day. It also freezes well.

TOTAL TIME: 1 HOUR 10 MINUTES

2 boxes (32 ounces each) low-sodium vegetable broth

2 leeks, trimmed and sliced, or 1 large onion, chopped

½ pound green beans, trimmed and snapped in half

½ pound carrots, cut into 1" lengths

1 can (14 ounces) fire-roasted diced tomatoes

1 teaspoon dried thyme

3 zucchini, sliced

2 cups cauliflower, cut into bite-size florets

Ground black pepper

In a large saucepan over medium-high heat, combine the broth, leeks or onion, and green beans and bring to a boil. Simmer rapidly for 10 minutes. Add the carrots, tomatoes, and thyme and let the soup return to a boil. Reduce the heat and simmer for 30 minutes.

Add the zucchini and cauliflower and simmer for 30 minutes, or until the vegetables are tender. Season to taste with pepper and serve hot.

Makes 8 servings

Chipotle, Orange, and Black Bean Soup

Chipotle provides this bean soup with a smoky kick, while the orange peel adds a touch of brightness. Be cautious with the chipotle. Its warmth and depth add great dimension to the soup, but too much can turn this from pleasantly hot to uncomfortably fiery. When I have fresh oregano, I use it in place of dried and stir it into the soup just before pureeing it.

TOTAL TIME: 30 MINUTES

2 teaspoons extra-virgin olive oil

2 shallots, chopped

2 cloves garlic, chopped

1 large carrot, chopped

1 canned chipotle chile pepper in adobo sauce, finely chopped

1 teaspoon ground cumin

1 teaspoon dried oregano

¼ teaspoon ground black pepper

¼ teaspoon sea salt

4 cups low-sodium vegetable broth

2½ cups cooked or canned black beans (rinsed and drained, if canned)

Grated peel of 1 orange

½ cup nonfat plain Greek yogurt (optional)

¼ cup chopped cilantro

In a large saucepan over medium heat, heat the oil. Cook the shallots, garlic, and carrot, stirring, for 3 minutes, or until the vegetables begin to soften. Stir in the chipotle pepper, cumin, oregano, black pepper, and salt and cook for 30 seconds. Add the broth, black beans, and orange peel (reserve a bit of the peel for garnish). Bring to a boil, reduce the heat to medium low, cover, and simmer for 15 minutes.

Transfer 2 cups of the soup to a blender and puree until smooth. Return the pureed soup to the pan and stir well. Ladle the soup into 4 soup bowls and serve with a dollop of yogurt (if desired) and a sprinkle of orange peel and cilantro.

Makes 4 servings

Roasted Vegetable and Strawberry Gazpacho

Roasting the tomatoes, zucchini, and bell pepper imparts a smoky flavor to the soup. It only gets better after resting for a day or two in the refrigerator. When serving cold soups, let the soup come to room temperature for about 15 minutes and then ladle it into chilled bowls. Chilled soups should be just that—chilled—not freezing cold. Garnish options include a dollop of pesto, goat cheese, chopped chives, diced avocado, and/or microgreens.

TOTAL TIME: 30 MINUTES + CHILLING TIME

3 large tomatoes, halved (1½ pounds)

1 zucchini, cut in half lengthwise and then in half lengthwise again

1 red bell pepper, quartered

3 tablespoons extra-virgin olive oil, divided

½ pint strawberries

½ cup water

3 radishes, chopped

½ cucumber, chopped

⅓ cup torn fresh basil leaves

2 scallions, sliced

1 clove garlic, minced

2 tablespoons red wine vinegar

½ teaspoon chipotle chile powder (optional)

½ teaspoon sea salt

¼ teaspoon ground black pepper

Preheat the oven to 425°F.

In an ovenproof dish, combine the tomatoes, zucchini, and bell pepper with 1 tablespoon of the oil. Roast the vegetables, turning them at least once, for 15 to 20 minutes, or until they are softened.

In a blender or food processor, combine the strawberries and water. Blend or process until smooth. Add the roasted vegetables, radishes, cucumber, basil, scallions, garlic, vinegar, chile powder (if desired), salt, black pepper, and the remaining 2 tablespoons oil. Pulse several times, or until the mixture is slightly chunky. Chill the soup for at least 2 hours before serving.

Makes 6 servings

Photo on page 116

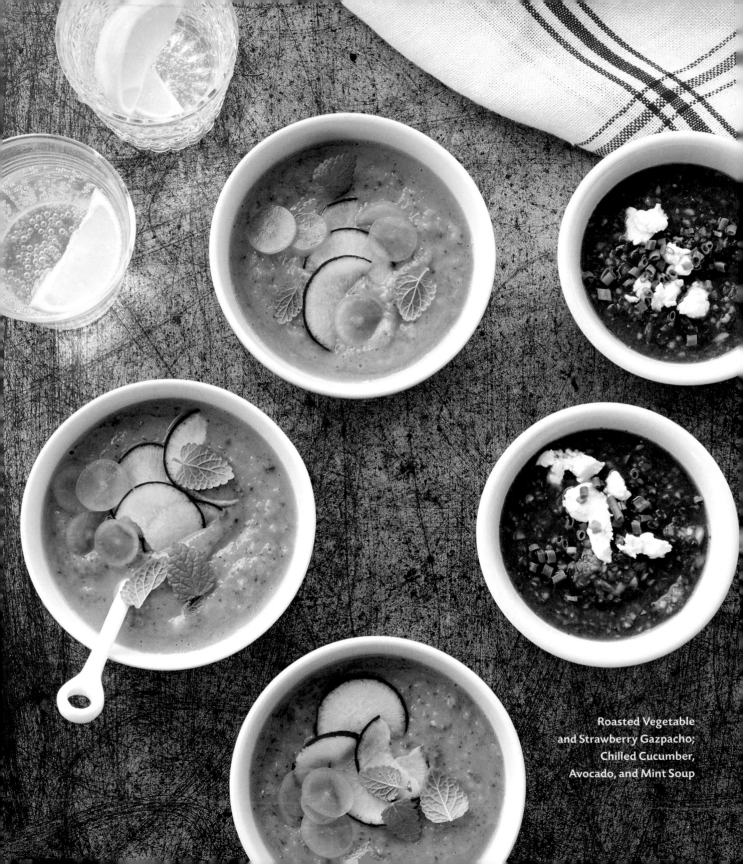

Roasted Vegetable
and Strawberry Gazpacho;
Chilled Cucumber,
Avocado, and Mint Soup

Chilled Cucumber, Avocado, and Mint Soup

Avocado gives this soup some creamy body, while the grapes lend sweetness. The soup will keep in the fridge for 3 days—just give it a good stir before serving.

TOTAL TIME: 15 MINUTES + CHILLING TIME

- 2 large cucumbers, halved lengthwise, seeds scooped out, and chopped
- 1½ cups green grapes + additional for garnish (optional)
- 1 small avocado, pitted and flesh scooped out + additional for garnish (optional)
- ⅓ cup fresh mint leaves + additional for garnish (optional)
- 2 scallions, chopped
- 1 clove garlic, chopped
- 1 small jalapeño chile pepper, seeded and finely chopped (wear plastic gloves when handling)
- Juice of 1 lime
- 2 tablespoons white wine vinegar
- ¼ teaspoon sea salt
- ¼ teaspoon ground white pepper
- ½ cup water
- Radish, for garnish (optional)

In a blender or food processor, combine the cucumbers, grapes, avocado, mint, scallions, garlic, jalapeño pepper, lime juice, vinegar, salt, white pepper, and water. Blend or process until smooth. Add more water if the soup is too thick, pulsing to mix. Chill the soup for at least 2 hours before serving.

Divide the soup among 6 soup bowls and garnish with thinly sliced radish and/or grapes and mint (if desired).

Makes 6 servings

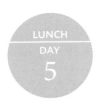

Vegetarian Chili

While this chili has a number of ingredients, once everything is chopped and measured, it quickly comes together. Beans are standard in vegetarian chilis, but eggplant is also used here for a "meaty" texture and flavor. A bit of cocoa calms down the heat from the peppers. There's plenty here to freeze for future meals.

TOTAL TIME: 40 MINUTES

1 tablespoon extra-virgin olive oil

1 yellow onion, chopped

1 pound cremini mushrooms, chopped

1 large yellow bell pepper, chopped

1 eggplant, chopped

3 cloves garlic, minced

1 canned chipotle chile pepper in adobo sauce, finely chopped

2 teaspoons ground coriander

1 teaspoon ground cumin

½ teaspoon sea salt

1½ cups low-sodium vegetable broth

4 plum tomatoes, chopped

1 can (14 ounces) black beans, rinsed and drained

1 can (14 ounces) red kidney beans, rinsed and drained

1 can (14 ounces) navy beans, rinsed and drained

1 tablespoon unsweetened cocoa powder

2 teaspoons dried oregano

1 small avocado, pitted, peeled, and sliced

⅓ cup chopped cilantro

In a large saucepan over medium heat, heat the oil. Cook the onion for 6 minutes, or until softened. Add the mushrooms, bell pepper, eggplant, and garlic and cook for 3 minutes. Add the chipotle pepper, coriander, cumin, and salt and cook, stirring, for 30 seconds. Add the broth, tomatoes, beans, cocoa, and oregano and stir to combine. Bring to a boil, reduce the heat, cover, and simmer for 20 minutes.

Divide the chili among 8 soup bowls and top with the avocado and cilantro.

Makes 8 servings

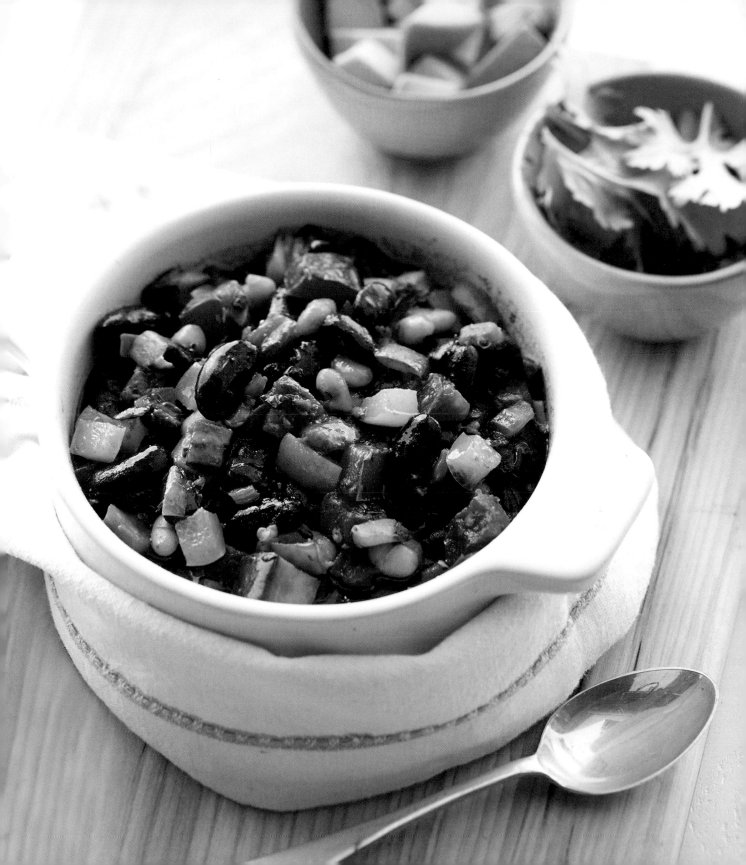

Turkey Chili

Turkey chili is a perfect make-ahead dish. The flavors only get better after it sits in the refrigerator for a day or two, and it freezes beautifully for last-minute meals. I like to garnish the chili with avocado or corn tortilla strips and a scattering of chopped cilantro. Want to add a touch of dairy? Top with a bit of sour cream, fat-free plain yogurt, or shredded Cheddar or Monterey Jack cheese.

TOTAL TIME: 45 MINUTES

1 tablespoon extra-virgin olive oil

1 pound lean ground turkey

1 yellow onion, chopped

1 large sweet potato, peeled and chopped

1 large red bell pepper, chopped

3 cloves garlic, minced

1 teaspoon ground cumin

½ teaspoon salt

¼ teaspoon ground black pepper

1 can (28 ounces) diced tomatoes

1 can (5½ ounces) tomato paste

2 cups cooked or canned red kidney beans (rinsed and drained, if canned)

1 can (4 ounces) chopped green chiles

1 teaspoon dried oregano or dried thyme

1 avocado, pitted, peeled, and chopped

In a large saucepan or skillet over medium heat, heat the oil. Cook the turkey, stirring, for 5 minutes, or until browned. Remove the turkey from the pan and set aside.

Add the onion to the pan and cook for 5 minutes, or until softened. Add the sweet potato, bell pepper, and garlic and cook for 3 minutes. Stir in the cumin, salt, and black pepper and cook for 30 seconds to heat through. Return the reserved turkey to the pan and add the tomatoes, tomato paste, kidney beans, chiles, and oregano or thyme. Increase the heat and bring to a boil. Reduce the heat to medium low, cover, and simmer for 25 minutes, or until the sweet potato is tender.

Divide the chili among 6 soup bowls and top with the avocado.

Makes 6 servings

Turkey and Avocado Sandwich

I realize everyone knows how to make a sandwich, but since this turkey and avocado sandwich is lunch on Day 1 (before you give up wheat), I want you to have the exact ingredients. Make your sandwich exceptional by using the best whole grain bread, ripe avocado and tomato, and a few slices of protein-rich turkey. Toast the bread for a satisfying crunch.

TOTAL TIME: 5 MINUTES

2 slices whole wheat or whole grain bread

2 leaves romaine lettuce

2 slices tomato

4 slices cucumber

¼ avocado, mashed

4 thin slices red onion

4 thin slices turkey breast

Spicy mustard (optional)

On 1 slice of bread, layer the vegetables and turkey in your favorite order. Spread the mustard (if desired) on the remaining slice of bread and place on top of the turkey.

Makes 1 serving

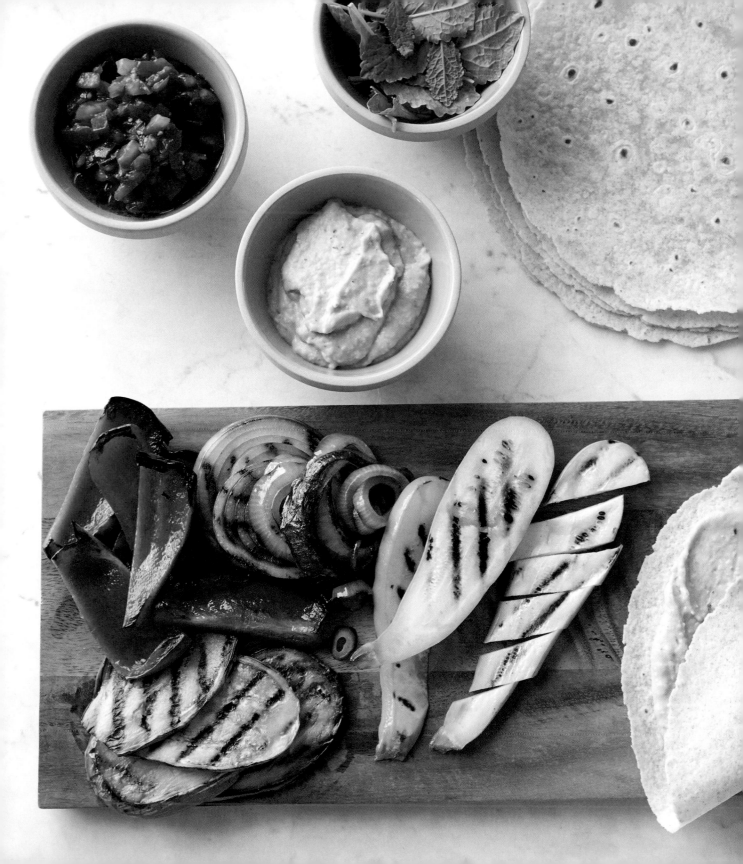

Grilled Vegetable Wraps with Roasted Garlic Bean Spread

VG WF GF DF

The zucchini, eggplant, bell pepper, and onion can be grilled outdoors or roasted in the oven at 400°F for 20 to 25 minutes.

Both the vegetables and the bean spread can be made and refrigerated up to 3 days in advance, but the wraps are best when prepared just before serving.

TOTAL TIME: ABOUT 1 HOUR

BEAN SPREAD

- 1 bulb garlic
- 3 tablespoons extra-virgin olive oil, divided
- 2 cups cooked or canned (rinsed and drained) navy beans
- 2 teaspoons fresh thyme leaves
- 1 teaspoon lemon peel
- Juice of ½ lemon
- ¼ teaspoon sea salt

WRAPS

- 1 zucchini or yellow summer squash, cut lengthwise into ¼" slices
- 1 eggplant, cut lengthwise into ¼" slices
- 1 large red bell pepper, quartered
- 1 small red onion, cut into ¼" rounds
- 1 tablespoon extra-virgin olive oil
- 4 large gluten-free bread wraps
- 2 cups baby kale or baby spinach
- Salsa

To make the bean spread: Preheat the oven to 375°F. Slice off about ½" from the top of the garlic bulb so most of the cloves are exposed. Drizzle the top with 1 teaspoon of the oil and wrap tightly in foil. Place the wrapped garlic in a baking dish and bake for 30 to 35 minutes, or until the garlic is soft and can be pierced with a knife. When cool enough to handle, squeeze the garlic pulp into a food processor container. Add the navy beans, remaining oil, thyme, lemon peel, lemon juice, and salt. Process until smooth. Remove to a bowl, cover, and refrigerate.

To make the vegetables: Preheat the grill. In a large bowl, toss the zucchini or squash, eggplant, pepper, and onion with the oil. Grill the vegetables, turning as necessary, for 8 to 10 minutes, or until they are tender and slightly charred. Each type of vegetable requires different amounts of grilling time, so remove them from the heat when they are done.

To make the wraps: Divide the bean spread over the surface of each wrap and top with an equal amount of the grilled vegetables, the kale or spinach, and some salsa. Roll tightly, tucking in the ends as you roll, and slice each wrap diagonally in half.

Makes 4 servings

Shrimp Summer Rolls with Almond Dipping Sauce

Once you get the hang of working with rice paper wrappers, you will be making these frequently. Rice paper wrappers are sold dried, but a quick soaking—just 10 seconds or so—in hot water makes them soft, pliable, and slightly chewy. If you've never worked with rice paper wrappers before, buy a few extra so you can practice. You'll find rice paper wrappers and sambal oelek in the Asian foods aisle.

TOTAL TIME: 45 MINUTES

DIPPING SAUCE

- ¼ cup unsalted almond butter
- 3 tablespoons unsweetened coconut milk
- 1 teaspoon grated fresh ginger
- 1 clove garlic, grated
- 1 tablespoon gluten-free soy sauce or tamari
- 1 tablespoon rice vinegar
- 2 teaspoons sambal oelek
- 1 teaspoon honey

ROLLS

- 3 cups water
- ½ pound large shrimp, peeled and deveined
- 12 rice paper wrappers (8" diameter)
- 2 cups shredded red cabbage
- 1 large carrot, grated
- 1 avocado, pitted, peeled, and thinly sliced
- 1 mango, pitted, peeled, and cut into strips
- ½ cup sliced fresh mint leaves

To make the dipping sauce: In a small bowl, whisk together the almond butter, coconut milk, ginger, garlic, soy sauce or tamari, vinegar, sambal oelek, and honey. Set aside.

To make the rolls: In a medium saucepan, bring the water to a boil. Add the shrimp and immediately remove the saucepan from the heat. Cover and let the shrimp poach for 3 minutes, or until opaque. With a slotted spoon, transfer the shrimp to a bowl of ice water and let them cool for 3 minutes. Drain the shrimp and cut each in half lengthwise.

Fill a shallow plate with hot water. Dip 1 wrapper in the hot water for 10 to 15 seconds, or until pliable. Taking care not to tear the wrapper, remove it from the water and spread it flat on a work surface. Place a little of the cabbage, carrot, avocado, mango, and mint on the bottom third of the wrapper (you will need one-twelfth of each ingredient per wrapper). Top with 4 pieces of shrimp. Fold the bottom of the rice paper over the filling and begin rolling tightly. Fold the left and right sides of the paper over the filling. Finish rolling tightly and slice in half diagonally. Repeat with the remaining wrappers and filling. Serve with the reserved dipping sauce.

Makes 6 servings

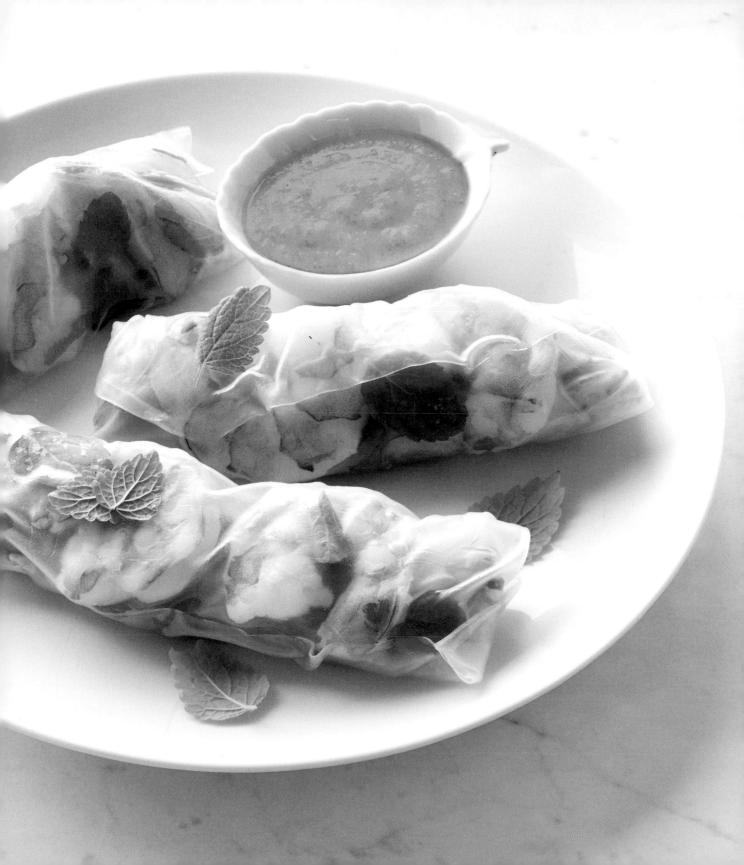

Collard Wraps with Tomato Hummus

Instead of making wraps with romaine or other lettuce leaves, try nutrient-rich collard greens. Be sure to cut off the white portion of the stalk from each leaf.

TOTAL TIME: 25 MINUTES

TOMATO HUMMUS

- 1 can (15 ounces) chickpeas, rinsed and drained
- ⅓ cup dry-packed sun-dried tomatoes
- 3 tablespoons tahini
- 2 tablespoons extra-virgin olive oil
- 2 cloves garlic, chopped
- 1 teaspoon smoked hot paprika
- 1 teaspoon grated lemon peel
  Juice of ½ lemon
- ¼ teaspoon sea salt

WRAPS

- 8 large collard green leaves
- 1 large yellow bell pepper, thinly sliced
- 1 zucchini, cut into matchsticks
- ⅓ cup fresh flat-leaf parsley

To make the tomato hummus: In a food processor, combine the chickpeas, tomatoes, tahini, oil, garlic, paprika, lemon peel, lemon juice, and salt. Process just until chunky.

To make the wraps: Cut the firm white stalks off the collards. With a sharp knife, slice off the thickest parts of the remaining stalks that run down the backside of the leaves. Put 2 collards on a work surface, head to foot (stalk ends at opposite ends) with the paler sides facing up. The leaves should overlap slightly. Spread ⅓ cup of the hummus lengthwise down the center. Top with one-quarter of the pepper, zucchini, and parsley. Tightly roll the leaves beginning from the bottom and tucking in the sides as you go. Cut in half on a bias. Repeat with the remaining ingredients.

Makes 4 servings

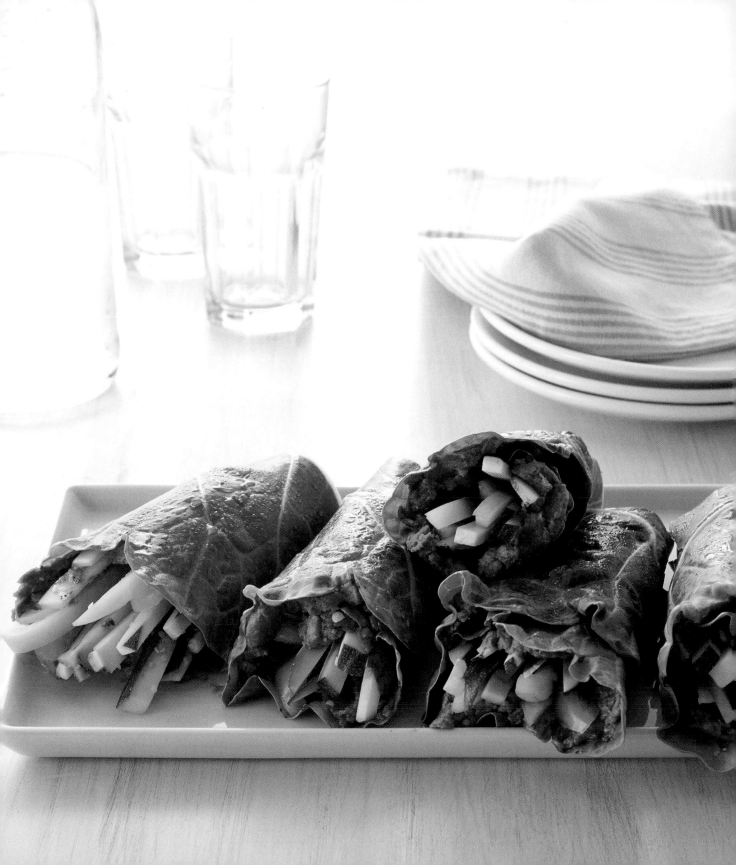

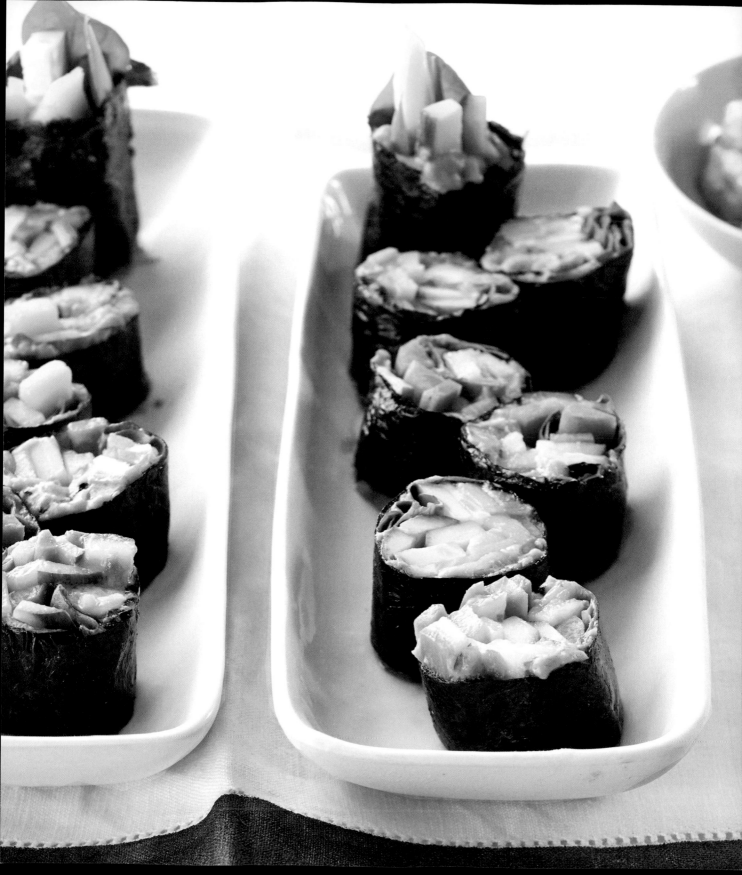

Nori Rolls with Avocado-Wasabi Sauce

Kids of all ages love to make Japanese rolls. Wait until they try their hands at these delicious bundles of salty nori, sweet mango, and matchstick vegetables. Remember, young ones might prefer less wasabi in the avocado sauce.

TOTAL TIME: 30 MINUTES

SAUCE

- 2 teaspoons wasabi powder
- 2 avocados, pitted and flesh scooped out
- Juice of 1 lemon
- 1 clove garlic, minced
- ½ teaspoon sea salt
- 2 tablespoons extra-virgin olive oil or avocado oil

ROLLS

- 8 nori sheets
- 2 carrots, cut into matchsticks
- 1 cucumber, cut into matchsticks
- 1 mango, pitted, peeled, and cut into matchsticks
- 2 cups baby spinach

In a small bowl, combine the wasabi powder and 2 teaspoons of cold water. Stir into a paste.

To make the sauce: In a blender or food processor, combine the avocados, wasabi paste, lemon juice, garlic, and salt. Blend or process until almost smooth. With the machine running, add the oil in a slow, steady stream, blending until the dressing is thick. Pour the dressing into a bowl.

To make the rolls: Lay a nori sheet, rough side up, on a cutting board. Spread 2 tablespoons of the avocado sauce onto the bottom half of the sheet. At the bottom edge of the sheet, arrange one-eighth of the carrots, cucumber, mango, and spinach. Fold the nori over the filling, and roll away from you as tightly as possible. Moisten the top edge of the sheet with a little water to seal the roll. Slice each roll into 8 pieces to serve. Repeat with the remaining ingredients.

Makes 8 servings

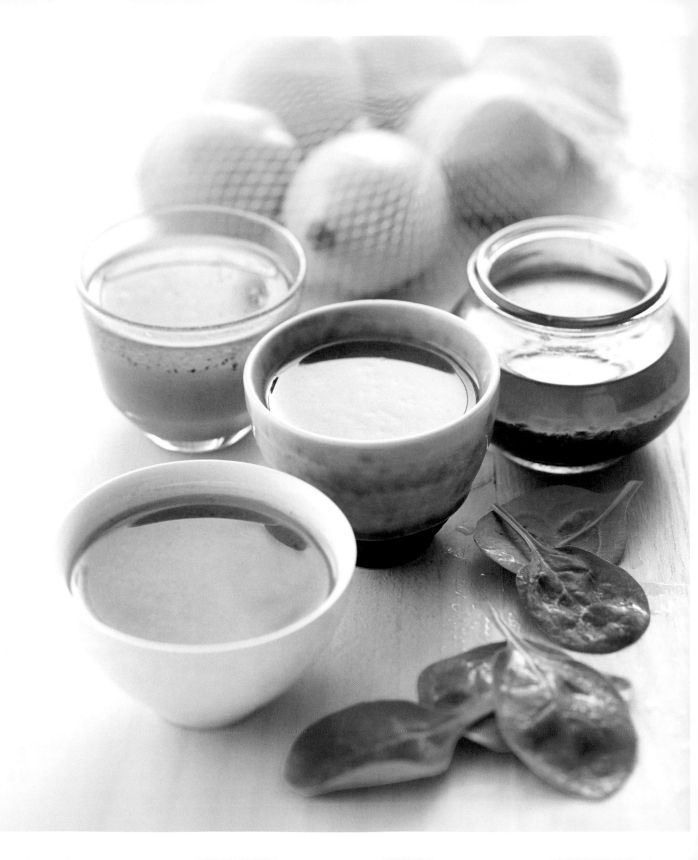

13

salads and dressings

Salads are one of the first things I developed
when creating the Healthy You Diet recipes.
I wanted something more satisfying than just
a pile of greens topped with a bland dressing.
By adding a lean protein—some grilled fish or
chicken—and a scoop of beans or quinoa,
I was able to turn boring salads into a meal
with varied tastes and textures. It's difficult
to pick a favorite, but my go-to salads are
Three-Bean Salad (page 136), Grilled Salmon
and Citrus Salad (page 151), and Red Quinoa
Salad with Black Beans and Avocado
(page 141).

Chickpea Salad with Lemon and Mint

My mom introduced me to chickpeas when I was a little girl by using plenty of them in every salad she made. Today, I'm always looking for new ways to use them in my own healthy cooking, whether in side salads or main course dishes. Since I always have chickpeas, bell peppers, cucumbers, and scallions on hand, this combination has become a favorite. Grilled shrimp, chicken, or salmon turns this into the perfect summer supper.

TOTAL TIME: 15 MINUTES + CHILLING TIME

1 can (15 ounces) chickpeas, rinsed and drained

3 scallions, finely chopped

1 cucumber, peeled, seeded, and chopped

½ red bell pepper, chopped

¼ cup chopped fresh mint leaves

3 tablespoons white wine vinegar

3 tablespoons lemon juice

2 tablespoons extra-virgin olive oil

1 clove garlic, minced

¼ teaspoon sea salt

Ground black pepper

In a medium bowl, mix together the chickpeas, scallions, cucumber, bell pepper, and mint.

In a small bowl, whisk together the vinegar, lemon juice, oil, garlic, and salt. Season to taste with black pepper. Pour the dressing over the chickpea mixture and toss well to combine. Cover and refrigerate for 30 minutes before serving.

Makes 2 servings

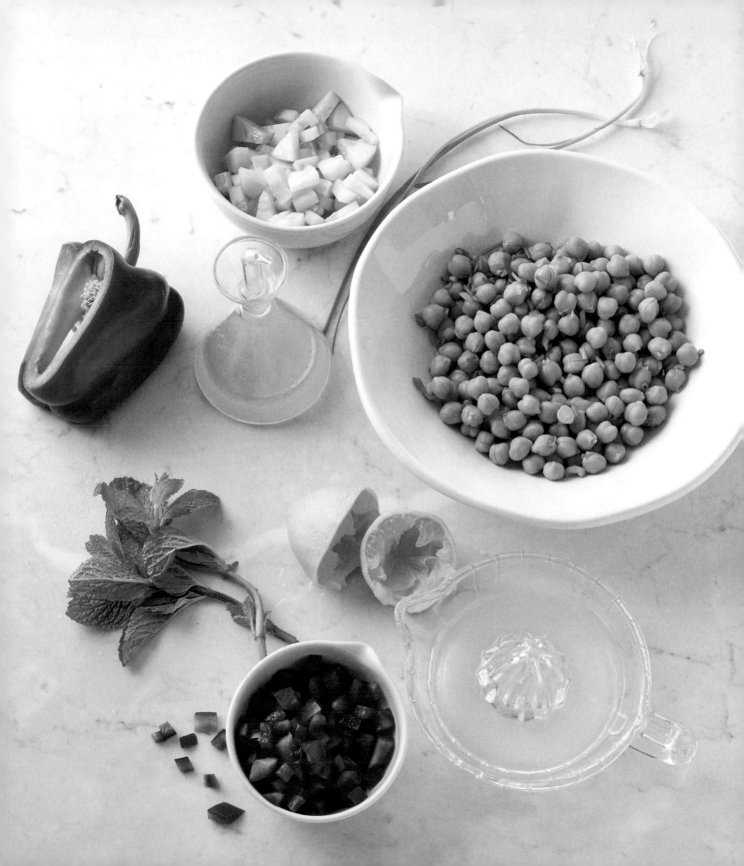

White Bean and Asparagus Salad

Green asparagus, white beans, and red and yellow grape tomatoes are combined to make this colorful yet simple salad.

TOTAL TIME: 15 MINUTES

1 bunch (12–16 spears) asparagus, trimmed and cut into 2" pieces

1 can (15 ounces) white beans, such as navy, rinsed and drained

6 grape tomatoes, halved

3 scallions, chopped

¼ cup chopped fresh flat-leaf parsley

¼ cup white balsamic vinegar

1 tablespoon extra-virgin olive oil

1 teaspoon Dijon mustard

¼ teaspoon sea salt

¼ teaspoon ground black pepper

In a medium saucepan with a steamer basket, bring 1" of water to a boil. Put the asparagus in the basket, cover, and steam for 3 to 5 minutes, or until tender. Do not overcook. Lift the asparagus from the steamer basket and let cool.

In a medium bowl, combine the beans, tomatoes, scallions, parsley, and cooled asparagus.

In a small bowl, whisk together the vinegar, oil, and mustard. Add the salt and pepper and whisk to combine. Pour the dressing over the bean salad and gently toss.

Makes 2 servings

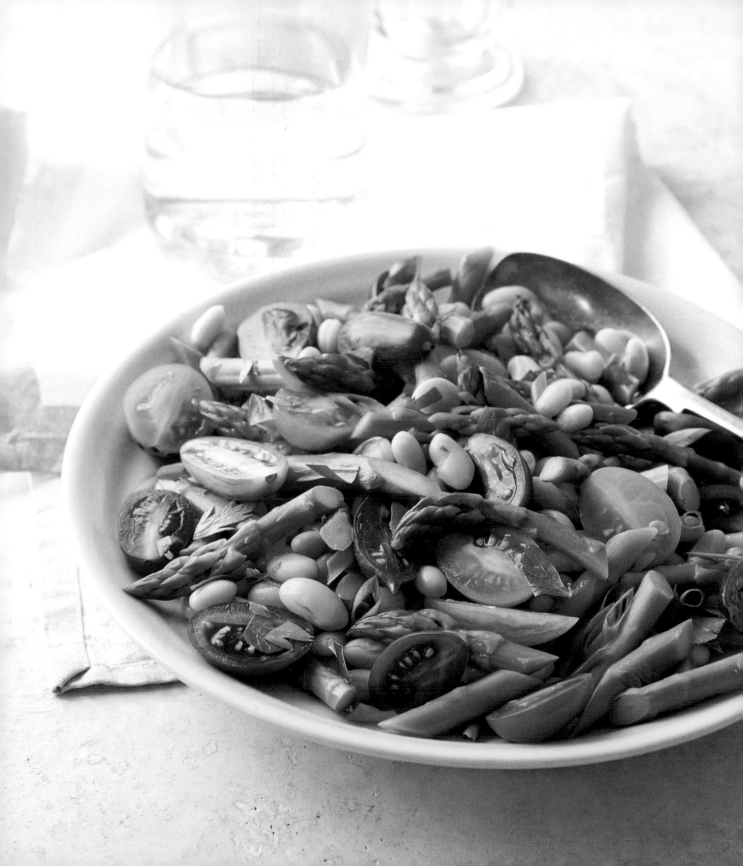

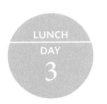

Three-Bean Salad

Nothing could be easier than opening 3 cans of beans and adding some vegetables and herbs for a quick salad. I often double this recipe because it tastes better after it sits for a day or two. My 5-year-old son eats it with tortilla chips. For lunch or as a party appetizer, I surround the salad with romaine lettuce or endive leaves, which can be used for scooping.

TOTAL TIME: 15 MINUTES + CHILLING TIME

- 1 can (15 ounces) white beans (such as cannellini), rinsed and drained
- 1 can (15 ounces) chickpeas, rinsed and drained
- 1 can (15 ounces) kidney beans, rinsed and drained
- 1 large tomato, chopped
- 2 ribs celery, finely chopped
- ½ red onion, finely chopped
- 2 tablespoons minced fresh flat-leaf parsley or cilantro
- ⅓ cup balsamic vinegar
- 2 tablespoons extra-virgin olive oil
- 1 clove garlic, minced (optional)
- ¼ teaspoon sea salt
- ¼ teaspoon ground black pepper
- 8–12 romaine lettuce leaves or 1 head Belgian endive

In a large bowl, combine the beans, tomato, celery, onion, and parsley or cilantro.

In a small bowl, whisk together the vinegar, oil, garlic (if using), salt, and pepper. Add the dressing to the beans and toss lightly. Serve immediately or store in the refrigerator for up to 3 days. This dish actually tastes better the next day. Serve with the romaine or endive leaves for scooping.

Makes 4 servings

Lentil-Carrot Salad

Warm lentil salad is a traditional French bistro dish, often served with lamb or other red meat. I make a lighter version and offer it warm, cold, or at room temperature on a bed of greens. Grilled salmon or a small piece of goat cheese makes this a main course.

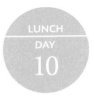

TOTAL TIME: 45 MINUTES

 2 cups green or brown lentils

 4 cups water

 2 bay leaves

   Sea salt

   Ground black pepper

 2 teaspoons extra-virgin olive oil

 4 carrots, chopped

 1 red onion, finely chopped

 1 clove garlic, minced

 3 tablespoons red wine vinegar

 2 tablespoons extra-virgin olive oil

 ¼ cup chopped fresh flat-leaf parsley

 1 cup coarsely torn arugula

 1 cup coarsely chopped Belgian endive

In a saucepan over medium-high heat, combine the lentils, water, and bay leaves and bring to a boil. Reduce the heat to low and gently simmer for 25 to 30 minutes, or until the lentils are tender. Drain, remove and discard the bay leaves, and transfer the lentils to a bowl. Season to taste with salt and pepper and set aside.

In a large skillet over medium heat, heat the oil. Cook the carrots, onion, and garlic, stirring frequently, for 4 to 5 minutes, or until the onion is translucent.

Add the carrot mixture to the reserved lentils and toss with the vinegar, oil, and parsley. Divide the arugula and endive among 4 plates and spoon the lentil salad on top of the greens. The lentil salad can be refrigerated for up to 3 days.

Makes 4 servings

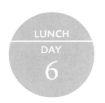

Pasta Salad with Vegetables

Because I don't want to live without pasta, I turn to rice pasta for some of my favorite dishes. Technically, rice is not a grain but a grass, so it is easier to digest. If you follow a gluten-free diet, brown rice pasta should have a place in it. I still eat wheat on occasion, although when I eliminate it, digestive issues disappear immediately. This recipe for pasta salad can be doubled easily, and just about any vegetables can be substituted for those I call for here.

TOTAL TIME: 20 MINUTES + CHILLING TIME

1 box (12 ounces) brown rice pasta, such as penne or fusilli

½ head broccoli, cut into small pieces

3 carrots, chopped

1 large tomato, chopped

3 scallions, finely chopped

2 teaspoons Italian seasoning blend

½ cup Italian Vinaigrette (page 161)

Prepare the pasta according to package directions.

In a medium saucepan with a steamer basket, bring 1" of water to a boil. Place the broccoli and carrots in the basket, cover, reduce the heat to low, and steam for 4 to 5 minutes, or until tender-crisp. Transfer the broccoli and carrots to a colander and run under cold water to stop the cooking.

In a large bowl, toss the pasta with the broccoli and carrots. Add the tomato, scallions, Italian seasoning, and vinaigrette and toss well. Cover and refrigerate for at least 1 hour before serving.

Makes 4 servings

Quinoa, Cranberry, and Almond Salad

LUNCH
DAY
7

Instead of the sugary cranberry relish traditionally served at Thanksgiving, I wanted to offer my family and guests a healthier version. Dried cranberries, sliced almonds, and fresh parsley make this a colorful addition to any holiday table. No dried cranberries or almonds? Then substitute raisins and walnuts.

TOTAL TIME: 20 MINUTES + CHILLING TIME

1 cup quinoa, rinsed and drained

2 cups water

½ cup chopped juice-sweetened dried cranberries

¼ cup toasted sliced almonds

3 tablespoons chopped fresh flat-leaf parsley

2 scallions, finely chopped

2 tablespoons lemon or lime juice

2 tablespoons extra-virgin olive oil

⅛ teaspoon sea salt

⅛ teaspoon ground black pepper

In a saucepan over medium-high heat, combine the quinoa and water and bring to a boil. Reduce the heat to low, cover, and cook for 15 minutes, or until the water is absorbed. Set aside, covered, to steam for 5 minutes. Fluff the quinoa with a fork and transfer to a bowl. Cover and refrigerate until chilled.

Add the cranberries, almonds, parsley, and scallions to the quinoa and toss to mix.

In a small bowl, whisk together the lemon or lime juice, oil, salt, and pepper. Pour the dressing over the quinoa mixture and toss well to combine. The salad can be stored in the refrigerator for 2 to 3 days.

Makes 4 servings

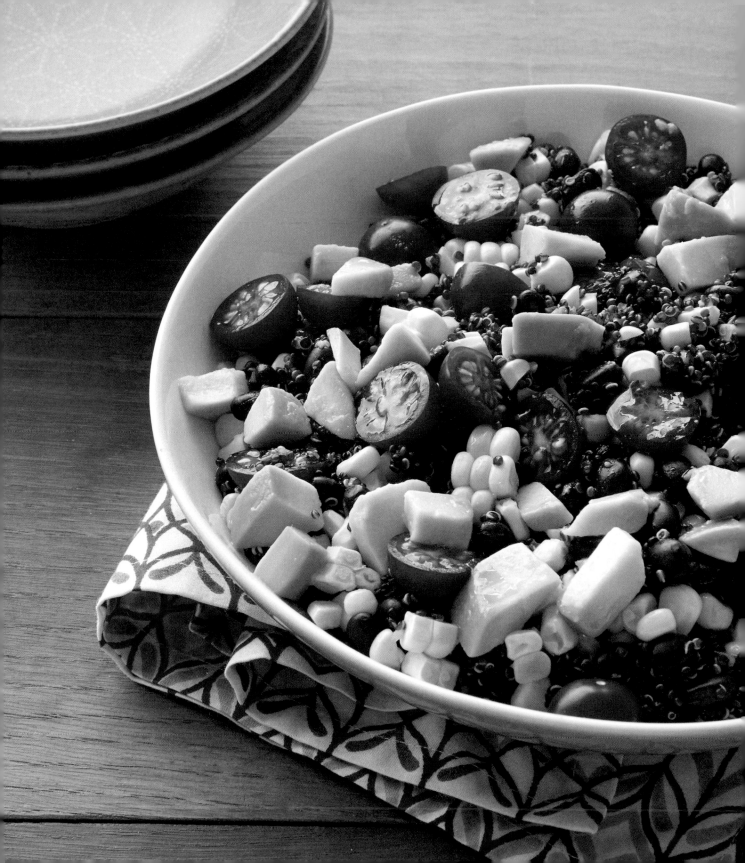

Red Quinoa Salad with Black Beans and Avocado

Wheat-free, gluten-free, high in protein, and low in calories, quinoa is one of the healthiest superfoods you can eat. This salad is so easy to prepare, you'll want to make it a staple in your healthy diet.

TOTAL TIME: 30 MINUTES + CHILLING TIME

  1 cup red or any other quinoa

  2 cups water

  2 tablespoons extra-virgin olive oil

  2 tablespoons lime juice

  ¼ teaspoon sea salt

  ¼ teaspoon ground black pepper

  1 cup fresh, frozen, or canned corn (thawed if using frozen)

  1 avocado, pitted, peeled, and diced

8–10 cherry tomatoes, halved

  1 can (15 ounces) black beans, rinsed and drained

In a saucepan over medium-high heat, combine the quinoa and water and bring to a boil. Reduce the heat to low, cover, and cook for 15 minutes, or until the water is absorbed. Set aside, covered, to steam for 5 minutes. Fluff the quinoa with a fork and transfer to a medium bowl. Cover and refrigerate until chilled.

In a small bowl, whisk together the oil, lime juice, salt, and pepper.

Add the corn, avocado, tomatoes, and beans to the quinoa and stir to combine. Add the dressing and stir gently. Cover and refrigerate for 30 minutes before serving.

Makes 4 servings

Quinoa, Egg, and Spinach Salad

There are any number of ways to personalize this chilled salad. Substitute arugula or kale for the spinach or add some diced cucumbers and summer squash along with fresh herbs of your choosing. The possibilities are endless. When I'm really busy or I don't want to wait for the quinoa to cool, a warm salad is just as tasty.

TOTAL TIME: 20 MINUTES + CHILLING TIME

½	cup quinoa, rinsed and drained
1	cup water
¼	cup white wine vinegar
2	tablespoons extra-virgin olive oil
¼	teaspoon salt
¼	teaspoon ground black pepper
2	cups baby spinach
8–10	cherry tomatoes, halved
2	large hard-cooked eggs, quartered

In a saucepan over medium-high heat, combine the quinoa and water and bring to a boil. Reduce the heat to low, cover, and cook for 15 minutes, or until the water is absorbed. Set aside, covered, to steam for 5 minutes. Fluff the quinoa with a fork and transfer to a bowl. Cover and refrigerate until chilled.

In a small bowl, whisk together the vinegar, oil, salt, and pepper.

Add the spinach and tomatoes to the quinoa. Add the dressing and toss until coated. Divide between 2 plates. Top with the eggs and serve.

Makes 2 servings

Clean Greens for Clean Eating

There's nothing worse than taking that first bite of a beautifully composed salad with greens or some sautéed spinach and finding yourself crunching on a few grains of sand. Since kale, spinach, Swiss chard, arugula, and lettuces are grown close to the ground in sandy soil, these greens need to be washed well before you use them. Even prewashed greens that come in clamshell containers should be cleaned.

Fill a sink or a very large bowl with cold water. Strip the thick stems from the greens' leaves and set them aside. Cut up the leaves as instructed in the recipe. In batches, add the leaves to the water and swirl them around well to loosen any dirt. Lift the leaves from the water, leaving any grit behind to fall to the bottom of the sink or bowl. Transfer the leaves to a colander or another bowl. Repeat, adding fresh water as needed, until the leaves are cleaned, then cut the stems as indicated in the recipe. If the greens are going to be cooked, don't dry them; the clinging water will turn to steam when heated. If the greens will be part of a salad, then dry them well with a paper towel or in a salad spinner.

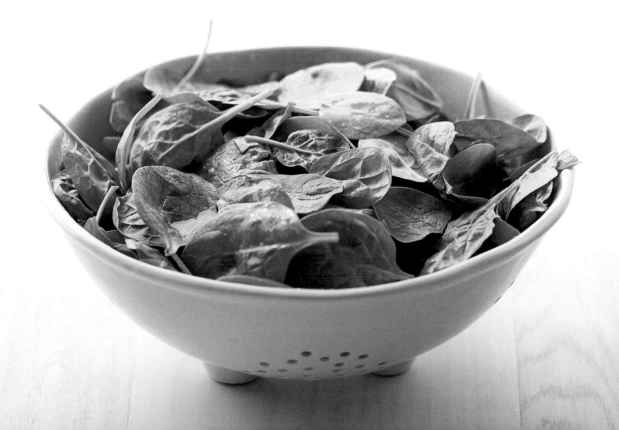

Quinoa, Tofu, and Vegetable Salad

While most people are familiar with tofu that has been grilled or stir-fried, it may come as a surprise that it also makes a delicious addition to chilled salads, especially on sultry summer days. Silken, or soft, tofu has a creamy, puddinglike consistency. Here, silken tofu is tossed with some vegetables and a vinaigrette for a quick meal.

TOTAL TIME: 20 MINUTES + CHILLING TIME

1 cup quinoa, rinsed and drained

2 cups water

Juice of 1 lemon

2 tablespoons extra-virgin olive oil

2 tablespoons white balsamic vinegar

¼ teaspoon sea salt

¼ teaspoon ground black pepper

½ pound silken tofu, cubed

12 cherry tomatoes, halved

½ red bell pepper, cut into matchsticks

4–6 scallions, chopped

4 cups baby spinach

In a saucepan over medium-high heat, combine the quinoa and water and bring to a boil. Reduce the heat to low, cover, and cook for 15 minutes, or until the water is absorbed. Set aside, covered, to steam for 5 minutes. Fluff the quinoa with a fork and transfer to a medium bowl. Cover and refrigerate until chilled.

In a small bowl, whisk together the lemon juice, oil, vinegar, salt, and black pepper.

Add the tofu, tomatoes, bell pepper, and scallions to the quinoa. Pour in three-quarters of the dressing and stir gently. Place the spinach in a salad bowl and scoop the quinoa salad on top. Drizzle the remaining dressing over the spinach leaves before serving.

Makes 4 servings

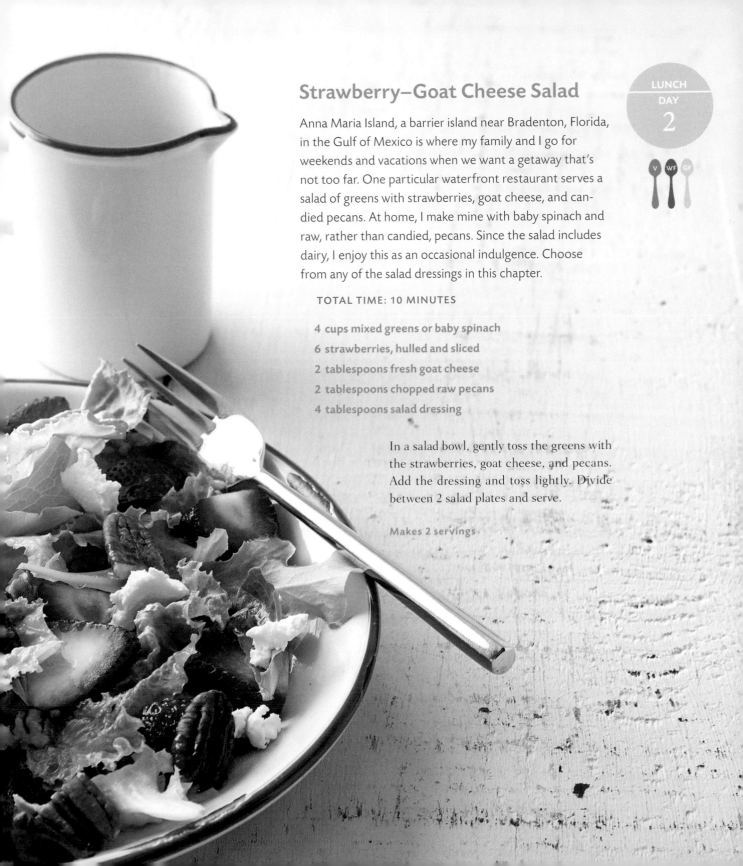

Strawberry–Goat Cheese Salad

Anna Maria Island, a barrier island near Bradenton, Florida, in the Gulf of Mexico is where my family and I go for weekends and vacations when we want a getaway that's not too far. One particular waterfront restaurant serves a salad of greens with strawberries, goat cheese, and candied pecans. At home, I make mine with baby spinach and raw, rather than candied, pecans. Since the salad includes dairy, I enjoy this as an occasional indulgence. Choose from any of the salad dressings in this chapter.

TOTAL TIME: 10 MINUTES

4 cups mixed greens or baby spinach

6 strawberries, hulled and sliced

2 tablespoons fresh goat cheese

2 tablespoons chopped raw pecans

4 tablespoons salad dressing

In a salad bowl, gently toss the greens with the strawberries, goat cheese, and pecans. Add the dressing and toss lightly. Divide between 2 salad plates and serve.

Makes 2 servings

Kale and Maple-Roasted Sweet Potato Salad with Walnut Vinaigrette

When lettuces and tomatoes are out of season, turn to this kale salad, which is topped with sweet potatoes, soft dates, and crunchy pumpkin seeds. Since kale can be tough and bitter, massage the leaves with the salad dressing for 30 seconds to 1 minute to soften them.

TOTAL TIME: 45 MINUTES

3 tablespoons pure maple syrup

1 tablespoon extra-virgin olive oil

1 tablespoon lemon juice

¼ teaspoon sea salt

2 sweet potatoes, cut into 1" cubes (1½ pounds)

⅓ cup pumpkin seeds

1 bunch curly-leaf kale, ribs removed, chopped

½ cup Walnut Vinaigrette (page 158)

½ cup pitted and sliced Medjool dates

Preheat the oven to 400°F. Line a baking sheet with parchment paper.

In a large bowl, whisk together the maple syrup, oil, lemon juice, and salt. Add the sweet potatoes and toss to coat with the maple syrup mixture. Spread the potatoes on the baking sheet and roast, stirring occasionally, for 30 minutes, or until tender. Remove from the oven and set aside to cool slightly.

In a skillet over medium heat, toast the pumpkin seeds for 2 minutes, or until they turn golden and begin to pop. Shake the pan often during toasting to make sure they don't burn. Transfer to a plate and set aside.

In a large bowl, toss the kale with the vinaigrette. With clean hands, massage the dressing into the kale for 1 minute.

Divide the kale among 4 serving plates and top with the reserved sweet potatoes, reserved pumpkin seeds, and dates.

Makes 4 servings

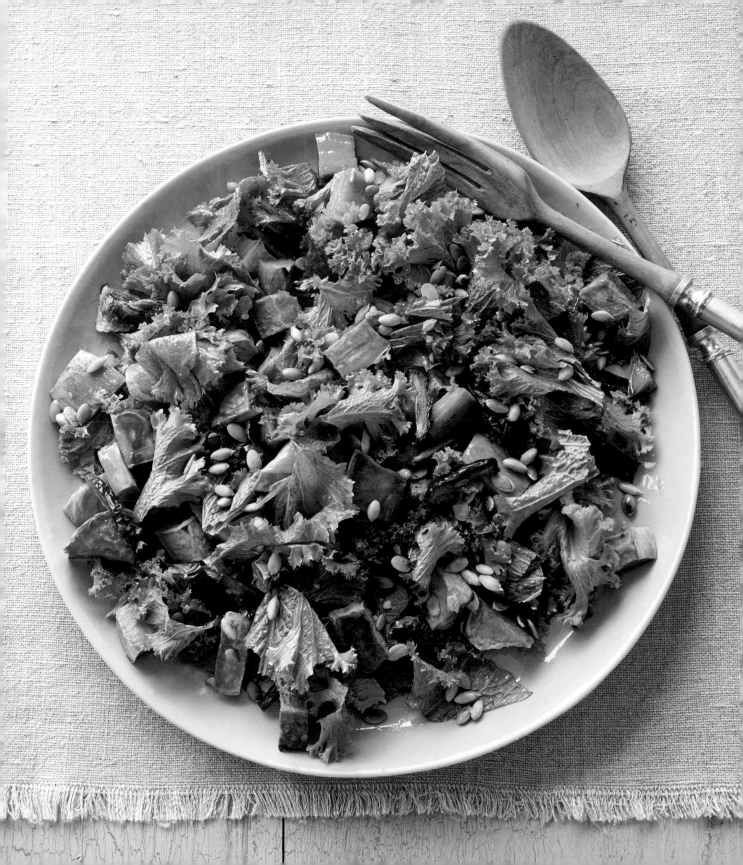

Chicken and Brussels Sprouts Slaw

In this delicious recipe, Brussels sprouts, a member of the cabbage family, are thinly sliced and used like cabbage in coleslaw. The shredding blade of a food processor makes quick work of the carrots, but you can also use the large holes on a box grater.

TOTAL TIME: 15 MINUTES

- 2 generous cups skinned, shredded rotisserie chicken
- ¾ pound Brussels sprouts, trimmed and thinly sliced
- 2 carrots, shredded
- 2 scallions, thinly sliced
- 1 large Granny Smith or Fuji apple, cored and cut into matchsticks
- ⅓ cup pomegranate seeds or juice-sweetened dried cherries
- ½ cup Maple-Hazelnut Vinaigrette (page 160)

In a large bowl, toss together the chicken, Brussels sprouts, carrots, scallions, and apple.

Divide the salad among 4 serving plates and sprinkle with the pomegranate seeds or cherries. Spoon on the dressing.

Makes 4 servings

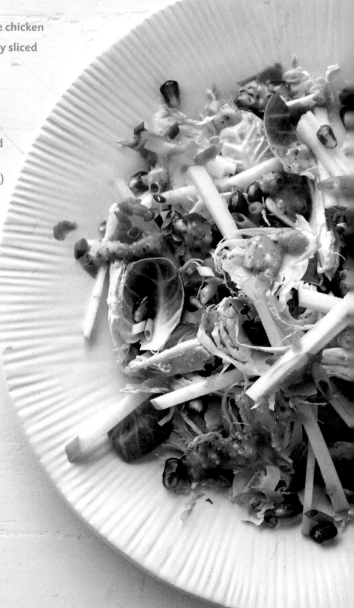

Chicken and Broccoli Rabe Salad

WF GF DF

Poaching chicken breasts in broth or water is quick and easy, but if you're short on time, purchase an already-cooked rotisserie chicken and use 2 cups of meat in the salad. Although I suggest tossing this salad with the Italian Vinaigrette, feel free to use any one of the Healthy You dressings in this chapter.

TOTAL TIME: 25 MINUTES

2 boneless, skinless chicken breasts (4 ounces each)

2 cups reduced-sodium chicken broth

1 bunch broccoli rabe, stems trimmed and leaves torn

1 can (15 ounces) white beans (such as cannellini), rinsed and drained

½ avocado, pitted, peeled, and cubed (optional)

6–10 grape tomatoes, halved

3 scallions, chopped

¼ cup chopped Italian parsley leaves

¼ cup Italian Vinaigrette (page 161)

In a medium saucepan, place the chicken breasts and cover completely with the broth. Bring the broth to a boil, then reduce to a simmer. Cover the saucepan with a lid and turn off the heat. Let the chicken breasts sit in the hot liquid for 10 to 12 minutes, or until cooked through. Transfer the chicken to a plate and set aside. Discard the broth.

In a medium steamer pan, bring 1" of water to a boil. Place the broccoli rabe in the basket, cover, and steam for 3 to 5 minutes, or until wilted and tender. Transfer the broccoli rabe to a bowl and let cool to room temperature. Add the beans, avocado (if desired), tomatoes, scallions, and parsley and mix well.

Divide the salad between 2 plates. Slice the reserved chicken breasts and arrange the slices over the salad. Spoon the vinaigrette over the salads.

Makes 2 servings

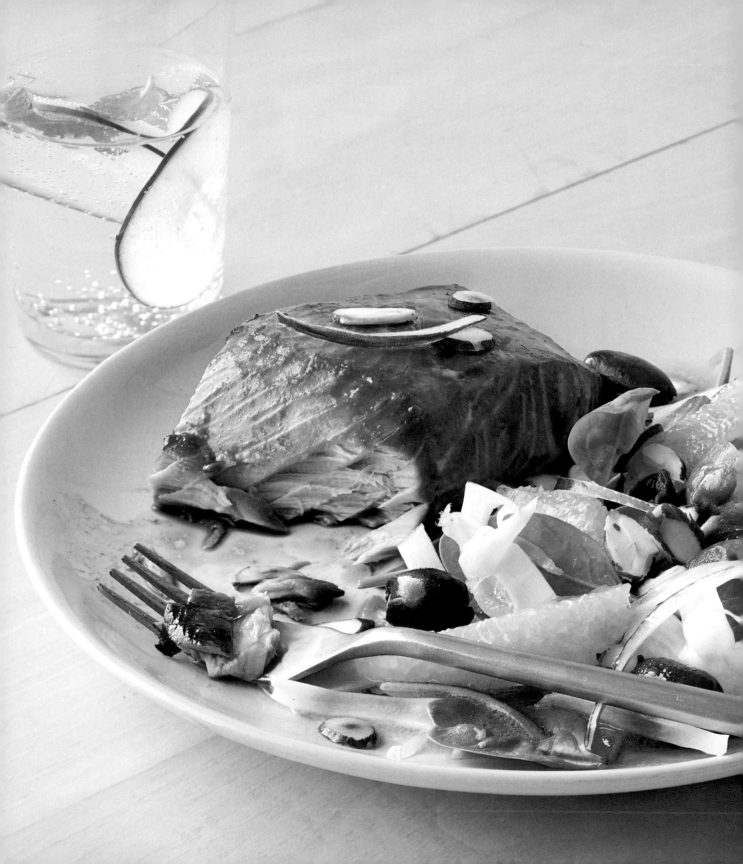

Grilled Salmon and Citrus Salad

When I don't have time to cook dinner and my pantry is empty, my family and I head to Bella Brava, my 7-year-old daughter's favorite restaurant in St. Petersburg. I like the grilled salmon salad with fennel and Florida citrus so much that I put my own spin on it and make it at home.

TOTAL TIME: 35 MINUTES

1 teaspoon honey

2 tablespoons gluten-free soy sauce or tamari

2 salmon fillets, skin removed (½ pound total)

1 teaspoon extra-virgin olive oil

3 cups baby spinach

½ fennel bulb, thinly sliced (optional)

Segments from ½ orange

Segments from ½ grapefruit

¼ cup thinly sliced red onion

1 tablespoon sliced almonds

4–6 kalamata olives (optional)

4 tablespoons Citrus Vinaigrette (page 163)

Preheat the broiler.

In a large resealable plastic bag, combine the honey and soy sauce or tamari. Add the salmon and shake gently to coat. Refrigerate for 10 to 15 minutes.

Lightly coat a broiler pan with extra-virgin olive oil. Remove the salmon from the bag and discard the marinade. Broil for 8 to 10 minutes, or until the fish is opaque.

In a medium bowl, combine the spinach, fennel (if desired), orange and grapefruit segments, onion, almonds, and olives (if desired). Divide the salad between 2 plates and top each with a piece of fish. Drizzle 2 tablespoons of vinaigrette over the fish and salad before serving.

Makes 2 servings

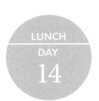

Crab, Mango, and Avocado Stacks

Ever wonder how chefs create perfect tall stacks of food for a dramatic presentation? Ring molds (open-ended cylinders) are the secret. Sure, you can arrange the crab, mango, and avocado on plates in a less constructed way, but layering the ingredients in ring molds is stunning and will make a splash at your next dinner party. Buy inexpensive ring molds at housewares stores, or you can use small tomato sauce cans, opened at both ends and thoroughly washed. Once you try this simple technique here, you'll be using it for other salads.

TOTAL TIME: 25 MINUTES

½ **pound jumbo lump crab, picked over**

1 **large tomato, chopped**

1 **cucumber, peeled, seeded, and chopped**

1 **mango, pitted, peeled, and chopped**

1 **avocado, pitted, peeled, and chopped**

2 **cups salad greens**

½ **cup Citrus Vinaigrette (page 163)**

Place the food ring mold or empty can on a salad plate. Press one-quarter of the crab into the mold, followed by a quarter of the tomato, cucumber, mango, and avocado. Press down on the food while slowly lifting the mold off the stack. Repeat with the remaining ingredients on separate plates.

Arrange the salad greens around each stack and drizzle with the vinaigrette before serving.

Makes 4 servings

Tuna Niçoise Salad

Although canned tuna is traditional for this classic French salad, I prefer fresh tuna that is pan-seared just until it's medium-rare. Boiled potatoes are also customary, but I roast them until tender on the inside and crisp on the outside.

TOTAL TIME: 35 MINUTES

SALAD

- 12 ounces new potatoes, quartered
- 4 teaspoons extra-virgin olive oil, divided
- ½ pound green beans, ends trimmed and halved crosswise
- 1 pound sushi-quality tuna
- Sea salt
- Ground black pepper
- 4 cups baby spinach
- 4 large hard-cooked eggs, quartered
- ½ English cucumber, thinly sliced
- 1½ cups halved grape tomatoes
- ⅓ cup pitted niçoise or kalamata olives, sliced
- 2 tablespoons chopped chives

DRESSING

- 1 tin (2 ounces) anchovies in olive oil, drained and finely chopped
- 2 tablespoons red wine vinegar
- 2 teaspoons minced fresh oregano (optional)
- 1 teaspoon Dijon mustard
- 1 clove garlic, minced
- ¼ cup extra-virgin olive oil
- Ground black pepper

Preheat the oven to 400°F.

To make the salad: In a bowl, toss the potatoes with 1 teaspoon of the oil and spread on a baking sheet. Roast for 30 minutes, or until crisp on the outside and tender in the center. Set aside.

Meanwhile, in a medium saucepan with a steamer basket, bring 1" of water to a boil. Place the green beans in the basket, cover, and steam for 4 to 6 minutes, or until tender. Set aside.

In a heavy skillet over medium-high heat, heat the remaining 3 teaspoons oil. Season the tuna on both sides with salt and pepper to taste. When the oil is shimmering, sear the tuna for 2 minutes, turning once, for medium-rare. Transfer to a cutting board to rest.

To make the dressing: In a small bowl, combine the anchovies, vinegar, oregano (if desired), mustard, and garlic. Whisk in the oil and season with pepper to taste.

Place the salad greens on 4 plates and arrange the reserved potatoes, reserved green beans, eggs, cucumber, tomatoes, and olives over them. Slice the tuna into ¼"-thick slices and divide among the plates. Drizzle the salad with the dressing and garnish with the chives.

Makes 4 servings

Sesame-Crusted Ahi Tuna and Cucumber-Seaweed Salad

Cucumber-seaweed salad is a popular dish in Japanese cuisine. You can find packages of dried wakame at most natural food stores and Asian markets. If wasabi paste is unavailable and you still want some fiery kick, stir in a pinch of red-pepper flakes. While black and white sesame seeds lend a visually pleasing touch, use only the white ones if that's all you have.

TOTAL TIME: 25 MINUTES

SALAD

- ½ ounce dried wakame
- 1 English cucumber, thinly sliced
- 4 radishes, thinly sliced
- 2 scallions, thinly sliced
- 2 tablespoons rice vinegar
- 1 tablespoon gluten-free soy sauce or tamari
- 2 teaspoons toasted sesame oil
- 1 teaspoon honey
- 1 teaspoon grated or finely minced fresh ginger
- 1 teaspoon wasabi paste (optional)

AHI TUNA

- ½ cup white sesame seeds
- ¼ cup black sesame seeds
- 4 ahi tuna steaks (1½ pounds total)
  Sea salt
  Ground black pepper
- 2 tablespoons peanut oil

To make the salad: In a bowl, cover the wakame with cold water and let it sit for approximately 15 minutes, or until fully hydrated. Drain, squeeze out the excess water, and slice into 2" pieces, if necessary.

In a large bowl, combine the cucumber, radishes, scallions, and wakame. In a small bowl, whisk together the vinegar, soy sauce or tamari, sesame oil, honey, ginger, and wasabi paste (if desired). Add the dressing to the cucumber salad and toss.

To make the tuna: In a shallow dish, stir together the white and black sesame seeds. Season the tuna with salt and pepper to taste and pat the sesame seeds on both sides of the tuna.

In a heavy skillet over medium-high heat, heat the oil until it shimmers. Cook the tuna for 1 minute, or until the undersides of the white sesame seeds start to turn golden. Turn the tuna and cook for 1 minute for medium-rare, or until the undersides of the white sesame seeds again start to turn golden. Transfer to a cutting board and cut into ¼"-thick slices. Divide the tuna slices and cucumber salad among 4 serving plates.

Makes 4 servings

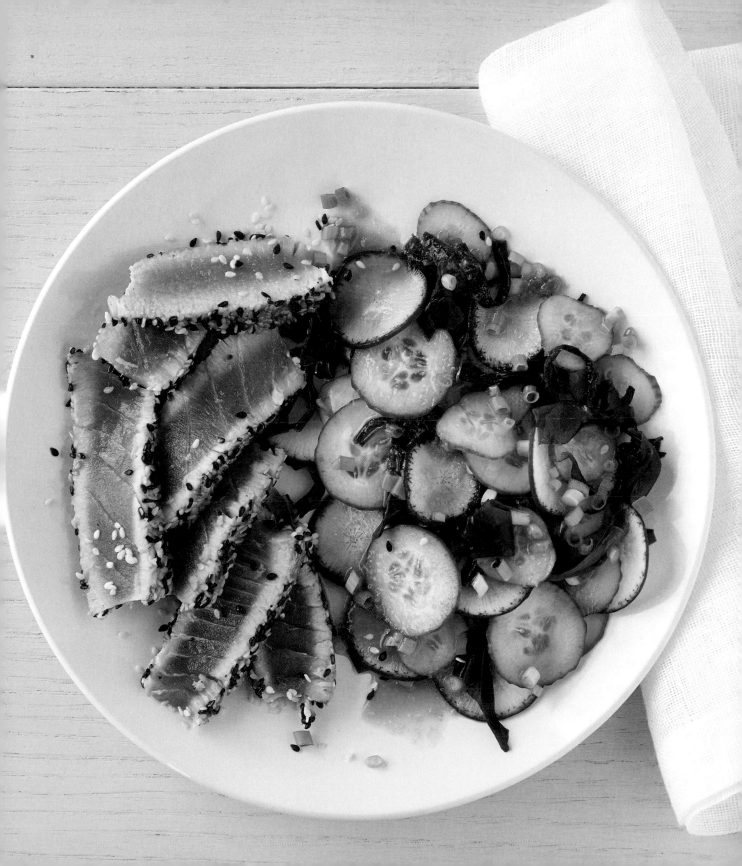

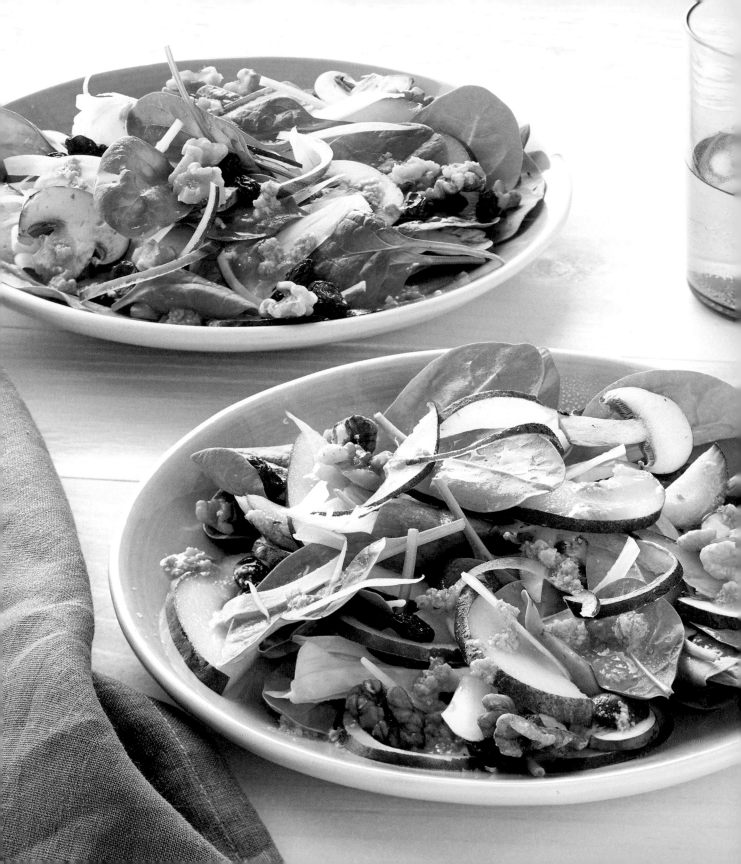

Spinach, Pear, and Walnut Salad

A sliced pear and walnuts put a new spin on the classic salad combination of spinach, mushrooms, and red onion. When drizzled with some Walnut Vinaigrette, this salad gives you a double dose of nutty goodness.

TOTAL TIME: 15 MINUTES

4 cups baby spinach

½ fennel bulb, thinly sliced

1 pear, cored, peeled, and thinly sliced

¼ cup coarsely chopped walnuts

¼ cup thinly sliced red onion

¼ cup sliced button mushrooms

2 tablespoons raisins

¼ cup Walnut Vinaigrette (page 158)

In a salad bowl, combine the spinach, fennel, pear, walnuts, onion, mushrooms, and raisins. Add the vinaigrette and toss just before serving.

Makes 2 servings

Walnut Vinaigrette

Drizzle this dressing with its little bits of walnuts over roasted or steamed vegetables, such as carrots and Brussels sprouts.

TOTAL TIME: 5 MINUTES

¼ cup extra-virgin olive oil

¼ cup walnut pieces

2 tablespoons apple cider vinegar

1 teaspoon Dijon mustard

1 teaspoon grated orange peel

1 clove garlic, chopped

¼ teaspoon sea salt

¼ teaspoon ground black pepper

In a blender or mini food processor, combine the oil, walnuts, vinegar, mustard, orange peel, garlic, salt, and pepper. Blend or process just until coarse.

Refrigerate any leftover dressing for 3 to 5 days. Shake well before serving.

Makes ½ cup

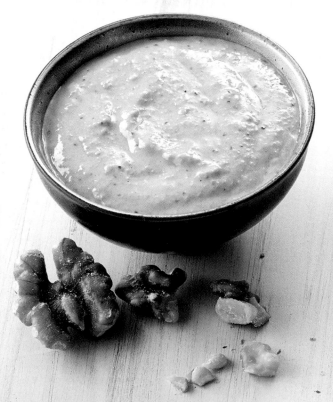

White Balsamic Vinaigrette

White balsamic vinegar is lighter in flavor than the dark variety. I prefer to use white balsamic vinegar when I don't want to add a dark color to salads and other dishes.

TOTAL TIME: 5 MINUTES

¾ cup white balsamic vinegar

¼ cup extra-virgin olive oil

2 tablespoons Dijon mustard

½ teaspoon sea salt

¼ teaspoon ground black pepper

In a jar with a lid, mix together the vinegar, oil, and mustard. Add the salt and pepper, cover with the lid, and shake well before serving.

Refrigerate any leftover dressing for 3 to 5 days.

Makes about 1 cup

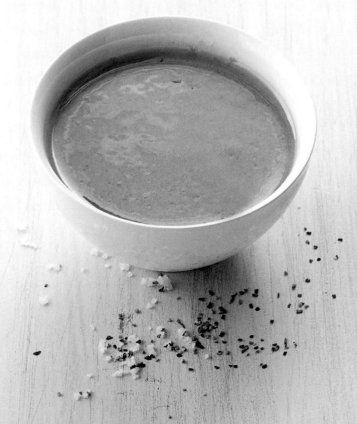

Maple-Hazelnut Vinaigrette

Like other nut oils, a small amount of hazelnut oil adds a distinct flavor to dressings.

TOTAL TIME: 5 MINUTES

¼ cup hazelnuts

3 tablespoons hazelnut oil or extra-virgin olive oil

2 tablespoons apple cider vinegar

2 tablespoons pure maple syrup

2 teaspoons Dijon mustard

1 teaspoon grated lemon peel

1 clove garlic, chopped

¼ teaspoon sea salt

¼ teaspoon ground black pepper

In a blender or food processor, combine the hazelnuts, oil, vinegar, maple syrup, mustard, lemon peel, garlic, salt, and pepper. Blend or process just until coarse.

Refrigerate any leftover dressing for 3 to 5 days. Shake well before serving.

Makes ½ cup

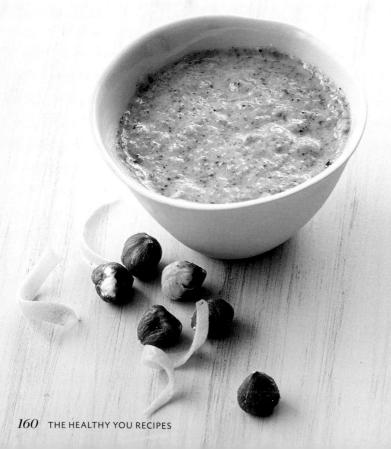

Italian Vinaigrette

Red wine vinegar gives this dressing a bit of bite. Spoon it over salads and grilled vegetables.

TOTAL TIME: 5 MINUTES

- 6 tablespoons extra-virgin olive oil
- 6 tablespoons red wine vinegar
- 2 tablespoons lemon juice
- 2 teaspoons Dijon mustard
- 2 teaspoons minced garlic
- ½ teaspoon sea salt
- ¼ teaspoon ground black pepper

In a jar with a lid, mix together the oil, vinegar, and lemon juice. Add the mustard, garlic, salt, and pepper. Cover with the lid and shake well before serving.

Refrigerate any leftover dressing for 3 to 5 days.

Makes about ¾ cup

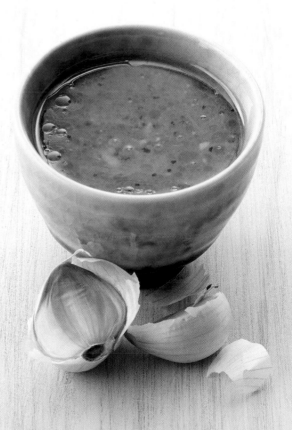

Greek Dressing

Oregano is what makes this vinaigrette so unique. While you can use dried oregano, I prefer fresh, which is available in markets year-round or from your garden in season.

TOTAL TIME: 5 MINUTES

½ **cup extra-virgin olive oil**

¼ **cup red wine vinegar**

¼ **cup lemon juice**

2 **tablespoons + 2 teaspoons fresh oregano leaves or 4 teaspoons dried oregano**

½ **teaspoon sea salt**

¼ **teaspoon ground black pepper**

In a jar with a lid, mix together the oil, vinegar, and lemon juice. Add the oregano, salt, and pepper. Cover with the lid and shake well before serving.

Refrigerate any leftover dressing for 3 to 5 days.

Makes about 1 cup

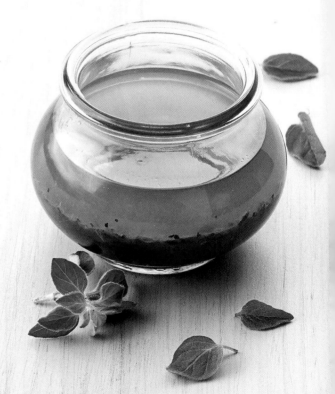

Citrus Vinaigrette

Drizzle this dressing over grilled fish, shrimp, or chicken for a bright flavor.

TOTAL TIME: 5 MINUTES

6 tablespoons red wine vinegar

¼ cup lemon juice

¼ cup orange juice

¼ cup extra-virgin olive oil

2 tablespoons Dijon mustard

½ teaspoon sea salt

¼ teaspoon ground black pepper

In a jar with a lid, mix together the vinegar, lemon and orange juices, and oil. Add the mustard, salt, and pepper. Cover with the lid and shake well before serving.

Refrigerate any leftover dressing for 3 to 5 days.

Makes about 1 cup

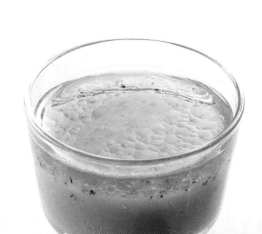

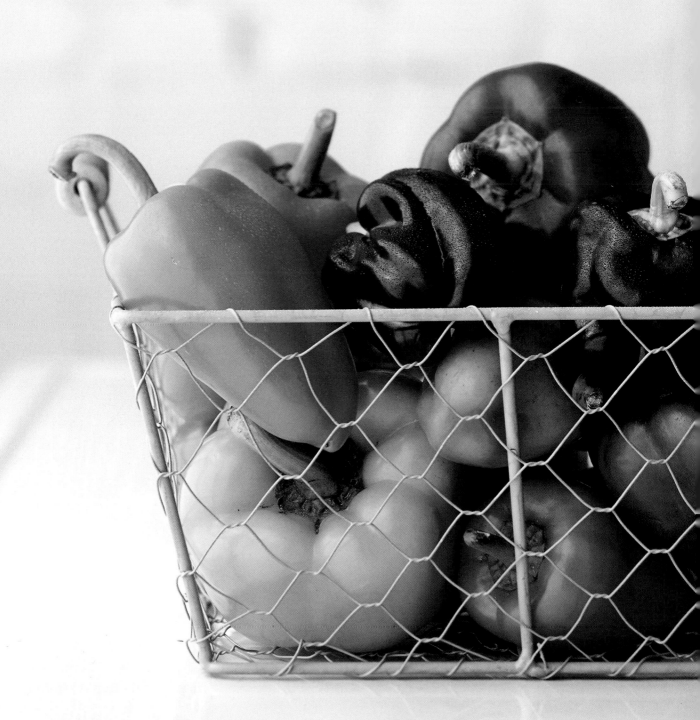

chapter

14

main meals

These main meal recipes provide you with a
variety of options so you're never bored with
the same-old, same-old dishes. Best of all,
there's plenty of great food here so everyone
can share, including Miso-Glazed Salmon
with Bok Choy (page 173), Crab Cakes
(page 195), and Black Bean Tostadas with
Salsa (page 197). There won't be any of that
I'm-on-a-diet-and-have-to-eat-something-
plain apology at the table. For oohs and aahs
at the table, definitely prepare the Snapper
and Asparagus en Papillote (page 174)—
moist fish gently oven baked in parchment
paper.

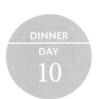

DINNER
DAY
10

Rosemary Chicken and Wild Rice

Chicken, rosemary, and garlic are a classic combination. In this recipe, the chicken breasts are quickly cooked on top of the stove, making this dinner an easy task. Start the wild rice first since it takes time to cook.

TOTAL TIME: 1 HOUR

2½ cups water

¾ cup uncooked wild rice

1 teaspoon extra-virgin olive oil

4 boneless, skinless chicken breasts, cut into 1"-wide strips

  Sea salt

  Ground black pepper

2 cloves garlic, minced

1 tablespoon chopped fresh rosemary leaves

1 tablespoon agave nectar or honey

1 tablespoon Dijon mustard

In a saucepan over medium-high heat, bring the water to a boil. Stir in the rice, reduce the heat, cover, and simmer gently for 40 to 45 minutes, or until the kernels puff open. Fluff the rice with a fork and simmer for 5 minutes. Drain any excess liquid from the pan and set aside.

In a large skillet over medium-high heat, heat the oil. Season the chicken with salt, pepper, garlic, and rosemary. Cook the chicken for 6 to 8 minutes, turning the chicken once, or until the chicken is no longer pink and the juices run clear.

Add the agave or honey, mustard, and reserved rice to the skillet and cook, stirring occasionally, for 2 to 3 minutes to coat the chicken and rice thoroughly.

Makes 4 servings

Grilled Herb Chicken

The chicken is mixed with herbs and garlic before it's cooked in a grill pan. Because there's oil in the marinade, the grill pan needs no oiling that day. The chicken, which is pounded to an even thickness, cooks quickly. If you're short on time, the chicken and marinade can be prepared and refrigerated up to 4 hours before grilling.

TOTAL TIME: 20 MINUTES

4 boneless, skinless chicken breast halves, pounded to an even thickness

1 tablespoon extra-virgin olive oil

1 teaspoon dried oregano

1 teaspoon fresh thyme leaves or ¼ teaspoon dried

1 teaspoon fresh rosemary leaves

½ teaspoon sea salt

¼ teaspoon minced garlic

Preheat a grill pan over medium heat.

Meanwhile, in a resealable plastic bag, combine the chicken, oil, oregano, thyme, rosemary, salt, and garlic. Shake the sealed bag to coat the chicken. Transfer the chicken to the grill pan and cook, turning once, for 6 to 8 minutes, or until a thermometer inserted in the center registers 165°F and the juices run clear.

Transfer the chicken to a serving platter and let it stand for 3 minutes to reabsorb the juices before slicing and serving.

Makes 4 servings

Pan-Grilled Chicken Breasts

Boneless, skinless chicken breast halves are a boon to the busy cook looking for a delicious lean protein. There are a couple of tricks for cooking the chicken so it remains moist and juicy.

First, the chicken should be lightly pounded to an even thickness. Chicken breast halves from the market are usually plump in the middle and thinner on the edges. These thin edges can over-cook while the center remains unappetizingly raw. It is very simple to pound the chicken to even it out. Just put a breast half between 2 plastic bags or sheets of plastic wrap. Hit the thick part of the chicken with a flat meat pounder or rolling pin until the meat is about $\frac{1}{2}$ inch thick. The pounded chicken will cook more efficiently and in less time. Or you can nicely ask the butcher to do it for you.

Avoid purchasing individually prepared and wrapped chicken breast portions. These may be convenient, but they are often injected with extra sodium-seasoned water to provide additional moisture.

When cooking chicken breasts, I use a ridged stovetop grill pan. It is much more efficient than a broiler (which heats up the kitchen) or an outdoor grill (which takes time to heat, and not everyone has one).

To cook boneless, skinless chicken breast halves, use a brush to lightly oil the pan. (I like the silicone brushes, which can go right into the dishwasher.) Preheat the pan over medium heat. Season the pounded chicken as directed in the recipe. Without crowding, add the chicken to the pan. Cook until the underside is lightly browned and seared with grill marks, 3 to 4 minutes. Using tongs, turn the chicken over and grill it for 3 to 4 minutes. Remove the chicken from the pan and let it stand for about 3 minutes to reabsorb its juices before slicing and serving.

Chicken and Vegetable Stir-Fry

This stir-fry makes for the perfect weeknight meal. For variety, add mushrooms, bell peppers, and other vegetables to the mix. The secret to a successful stir-fry is to make sure all of the vegetables are cut approximately the same size for even cooking.

TOTAL TIME: 1 HOUR

2½ cups water

1 cup uncooked brown rice

¼ cup low-sodium chicken broth

2 tablespoons gluten-free soy sauce or tamari

1 teaspoon vegetable oil

4 boneless, skinless chicken breast halves, sliced into ¼" strips

1 tablespoon minced garlic

2 teaspoons grated fresh ginger

2 cups broccoli florets

1 cup snap or snow peas

½ cup chopped carrots

2 cups baby spinach

1 cup bean sprouts

3 scallions, chopped

In a saucepan over medium-high heat, bring the water to a boil. Stir in the rice, reduce the heat, cover, and simmer gently for 40 to 45 minutes, or until the kernels puff open. Fluff the rice with a fork and simmer for 5 minutes. Drain any excess liquid from the pan and set aside.

Meanwhile, in a small bowl, whisk together the broth and soy sauce or tamari. Set aside.

In a large skillet over medium-high heat, heat the oil and swirl the pan to coat. Cook the chicken, stirring, for 3 to 4 minutes, or until it browns and is partially cooked. Add the garlic and ginger and cook, stirring constantly, for 15 seconds. Add the broccoli, peas, and carrots and cook, stirring constantly, for 3 to 4 minutes, or until tender-crisp. Add the spinach, sprouts, scallions, and reserved broth mixture. Cook, stirring constantly, for 3 to 4 minutes, or until the spinach wilts and the chicken is no longer pink and the juices run clear.

Fluff the rice with a fork and divide it among 4 plates. Spoon the chicken mixture over the rice and serve.

Makes 4 servings

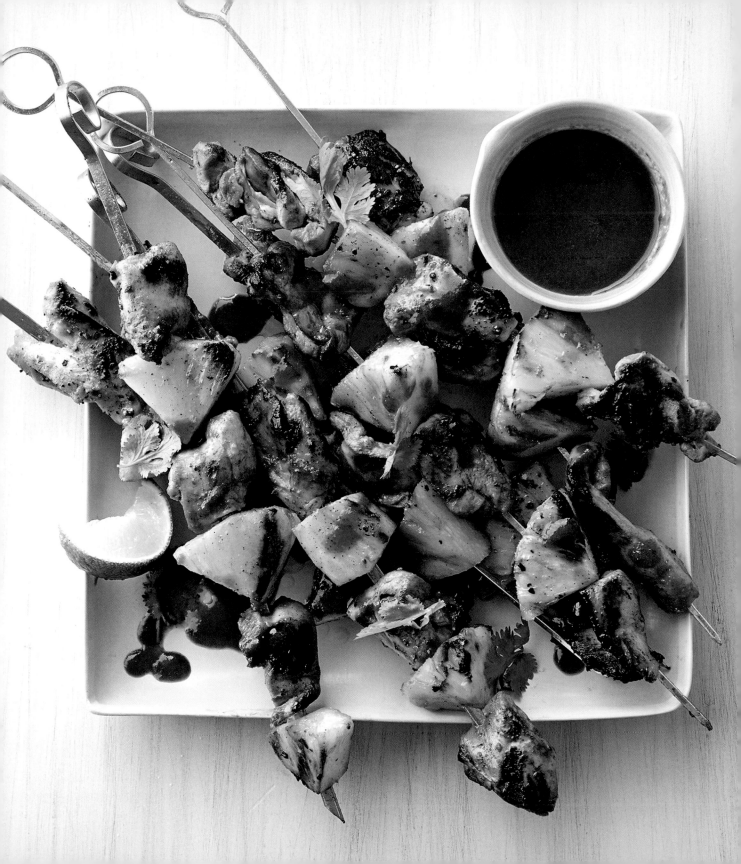

Chicken Skewers with Honey-Lime-Chile Sauce

When making chicken skewers, I find that chicken thighs are less prone to drying out on the grill. If using wooden skewers, soak them in water for 15 to 30 minutes so they don't burn on the grill.

TOTAL TIME: 30 MINUTES + MARINATING TIME

SAUCE

- 3 tablespoons honey
- 3 tablespoons gluten-free soy sauce or tamari
- 1½ tablespoons sambal oelek
- 1 tablespoon peanut oil
- Grated peel of 1 lime
- Juice of 2 limes
- 3 cloves garlic, chopped
- 1½" piece fresh ginger, chopped

CHICKEN

- 1 pound boneless, skinless chicken thighs, fat trimmed and cut into 2" pieces
- ½ pineapple, cut into 1" chunks
- Lime wedges (optional)
- Cilantro sprigs (optional)

To make the sauce: In a blender, combine the honey, soy sauce or tamari, sambal oelek, oil, lime peel, lime juice, garlic, and ginger. Blend until smooth. Remove ⅓ cup of the marinade to a small bowl, cover, and refrigerate until ready to serve as a sauce.

To make the chicken: In a bowl, combine the chicken and the remaining marinade. Toss well, cover, and refrigerate for at least 6 hours or overnight.

Preheat the grill to medium high. Alternately thread 2 pieces of chicken onto skewers, folding the pieces over if they are too long and thin, with 1 piece of pineapple until all of the chicken and pineapple has been used. Grill the skewers, covered, for 8 to 10 minutes, turning occasionally, or until the juices run clear. (Lower the heat or move the skewers to a cooler part of the grill if the chicken is browning too fast.) Transfer the skewers to a platter and drizzle with the reserved sauce. Garnish the platter with lime wedges and cilantro sprigs (if desired).

Makes 4 servings

DINNER

DAY

7

WF GF DF

Chicken Tacos

Who doesn't like chicken tacos topped with avocado, tomatoes, and a few drops of hot sauce? Kids never turn down tacos, making them a favorite weeknight supper. It's easy to roast the chicken, but if you prefer, grill it in a grill pan, as described on page 168.

TOTAL TIME: 30 MINUTES

TACO SEASONING

- 1 tablespoon chili powder
- 1 teaspoon ground cumin
- 1 teaspoon sea salt
- 1 teaspoon ground black pepper
- ¼ teaspoon garlic powder
- ¼ teaspoon onion powder
- ¼ teaspoon dried oregano
- ¼ teaspoon paprika
- ¼ teaspoon crushed red-pepper flakes (optional)

TACOS

- 4 boneless, skinless chicken breast halves, pounded to an even thickness
- 2 tablespoons Taco Seasoning
- ¼ cup lime juice
- 1 cup shredded romaine lettuce
- ½ cup chopped tomatoes
- 2 scallions, thinly sliced
- 1 avocado, pitted, peeled, and chopped
- 8 soft corn tortillas (6" diameter), warmed

  Hot sauce (optional)

Preheat the oven to 350°F.

To make the taco seasoning: In a small bowl, whisk together the chili powder, cumin, sea salt, black pepper, garlic powder, onion powder, oregano, paprika, and red-pepper flakes (if using) until combined. You can also put all of the ingredients in a jar, cover it, and shake it until they are combined. Store in an airtight container for up to 6 months.

To make the tacos: In a resealable plastic bag, combine the chicken and taco seasoning. Shake the sealed bag to coat the chicken with the seasoning.

In a baking dish large enough to hold the chicken in a single layer, pour the lime juice. Arrange the chicken in the dish and bake for 15 to 20 minutes, or until a thermometer inserted in the center registers 165°F and the juices run clear.

Let the chicken rest for 5 minutes before slicing into bite-size pieces. Divide the lettuce, tomatoes, scallions, avocado, and chicken among the tortillas. Serve with hot sauce on the side, if desired.

Makes 4 servings

Miso-Glazed Salmon with Bok Choy

DINNER
DAY
3

Rich, tender salmon stands up beautifully to a sweet-and-salty miso glaze. When teamed with wilted bok choy, it becomes a meal fit for guests. See page 107 for an explanation of the different kinds of miso.

TOTAL TIME: 30 MINUTES

2 tablespoons white or yellow miso paste

1½ tablespoons gluten-free, reduced-sodium soy sauce or tamari

1 tablespoon mirin or rice vinegar

2 teaspoons grated fresh ginger

2 teaspoons honey

4 center-cut salmon fillets (1½ pounds total)

2 pounds bok choy

2 teaspoons peanut oil

2 shallots, chopped

2 cloves garlic, chopped

Grated peel of 1 lemon

Juice of ½ lemon

Sea salt

2 teaspoons black sesame seeds

1 scallion, green part only, thinly sliced

Preheat the oven to 400°F.

In a small bowl, whisk together the miso, soy sauce or tamari, mirin or vinegar, ginger, and honey. On a baking sheet lined with parchment paper, arrange the salmon and brush with the miso mixture. Let the salmon stand for 10 minutes.

Bake the salmon for 10 minutes, or until opaque.

Meanwhile, separate the bok choy stems from the leaves. Slice the stems into thin strips and slice the leaves in half.

In a wok or large skillet over medium heat, heat the oil. Cook the sliced bok choy stems, shallots, and garlic for 3 minutes, or until the stems are tender. Stir in the bok choy leaves and lemon peel and cook just until the leaves wilt slightly. Remove from the heat, stir in the lemon juice, and season with salt to taste.

Place the salmon and bok choy on 4 plates and sprinkle with the sesame seeds and scallion.

Makes 4 servings

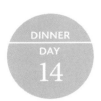

DINNER
DAY
14

WF GF DF

Snapper and Asparagus en Papillote

This is the final meal of the 14-day Healthy You Diet. What a way to end your 2 weeks! Enjoy every bite of this dish—you deserve it!

TOTAL TIME: 45 MINUTES

2½ cups water

¾ cup uncooked brown basmati rice

4 snapper or halibut fillets (1½ pounds total)

Sea salt

Ground black pepper

1 tablespoon extra-virgin olive oil

24 thin asparagus spears, trimmed

1 lemon, thinly sliced

2 tablespoons chopped fresh dill or flat-leaf parsley, or 1½ teaspoons dried dill

In a saucepan over medium-high heat, bring the water to a boil. Stir in the rice, reduce the heat, cover, and simmer gently for 40 to 45 minutes, or until the kernels puff open. Fluff the rice with a fork and simmer for 5 minutes. Drain any excess liquid from the pan and set aside.

Meanwhile, preheat the oven to 375°F.

Cut 4 sheets of parchment paper, each approximately 18" × 12". Fold the parchment in half the long way. Using scissors, cut a large heart out of each piece of paper, beginning the cut on the fold.

Season both sides of the fish lightly with salt and pepper. Place 1 fillet on one half of a parchment heart, leaving at least a 1" border. Drizzle with one-quarter of the oil and top with 6 asparagus spears and a few lemon slices. Sprinkle with one-quarter of the dill or parsley. Fold the other side of the heart over the fish and twist the edges together to make a seal. Fold the bottom edge under the packet to keep it from opening during cooking. Repeat with the remaining ingredients.

Transfer the packets to 2 baking sheets and bake for 12 to 15 minutes. Using oven mitts or tongs, transfer the packets to 4 plates. Be sure everyone is at the table to open their packet with scissors. Take care because the steam is hot. Serve with the rice.

Makes 4 servings

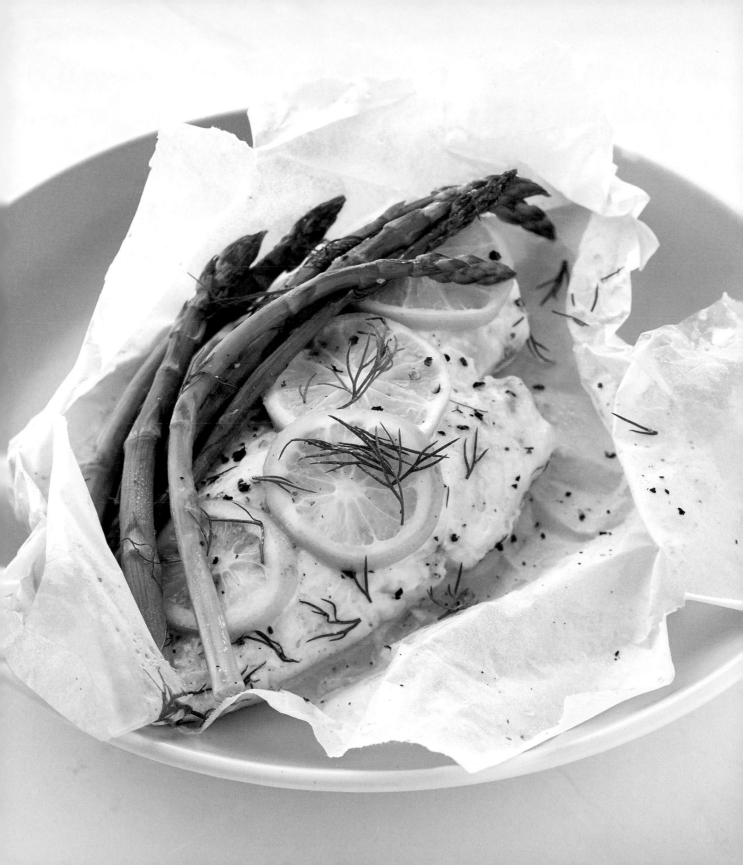

Steamed Sole with Butternut Squash Puree

Steaming fish results in moist fish without any added fat. It's a particularly quick and easy technique to use with delicate fish such as sole, but it works well with other fish, too. If you can't find sole, try steaming flounder, red snapper, or other thin whitefish. Many markets now sell peeled and cubed butternut squash.

TOTAL TIME: 25 MINUTES

2 teaspoons extra-virgin olive oil

1 leek, white and light green parts, thinly sliced

2 cloves garlic, sliced

3 cups peeled and cubed butternut squash

1 cup low-sodium chicken broth or vegetable broth

¼ teaspoon sea salt + more to taste

¼ teaspoon ground black pepper + more to taste

1 teaspoon grated lemon peel

4 sole fillets (1–1½ pounds total)

2 cups arugula

2 teaspoons balsamic vinegar

In a medium saucepan over medium heat, heat the oil. Cook the leek and garlic until the leek softens, about 3 minutes. Add the squash, broth, ¼ teaspoon salt, and ¼ teaspoon pepper. Bring to a boil, lower the heat, cover, and simmer for 15 minutes, or until the squash is tender. Transfer the mixture to a blender or food processor. Add the lemon peel and blend or process until smooth. The puree should be slightly thick. If too thin, strain through a fine-mesh sieve.

On a steamer tray lined with parchment paper, arrange the fish and season with salt and pepper. Steam over 2" of water for 7 minutes, or until it flakes easily.

Toss the arugula with the vinegar and salt and pepper to taste.

Spread the squash puree on 4 plates. Nestle the fish into the sauce and garnish with the arugula.

Makes 4 servings

Garlic Shrimp Pasta with Roasted Tomatoes

Shrimp, garlic, and pasta are a favorite combination. Add some roasted cherry tomatoes; roasting them emphasizes their inherent sweetness. Serve with a green salad tossed with Italian Vinaigrette (page 161) for a complete meal.

TOTAL TIME: 25 MINUTES

- 2 pints cherry tomatoes
- 5 teaspoons extra-virgin olive oil, divided
- Sea salt
- ¾ pound gluten-free brown rice pasta (such as spaghetti or linguine)
- ⅔ cup roughly chopped fresh flat-leaf parsley
- 3 cloves garlic, thinly sliced
- ¼ teaspoon red-pepper flakes
- 1 pound large shrimp, peeled and deveined
- Ground black pepper
- Juice of ½ lemon
- 2 tablespoons chopped chives

Preheat the oven to 400°F.

In a large bowl, toss the tomatoes with 2 teaspoons of the oil and a pinch of salt. Spread the tomatoes on a baking sheet and roast for 12 minutes, or until they begin to shrivel and are slightly collapsed.

Meanwhile, prepare the pasta according to package directions. Drain, return to the pot, and toss with the parsley.

In a large skillet over medium heat, heat the remaining 3 teaspoons oil until the oil shimmers. Cook the garlic and red-pepper flakes, stirring often, for 30 seconds, or until the garlic is fragrant and slightly golden. Add the shrimp and cook, stirring, for 2 to 3 minutes, or until opaque. Season with salt and black pepper to taste.

Divide the pasta among 4 plates and top with the shrimp and roasted tomatoes. Drizzle with the lemon juice and garnish with the chives.

Makes 4 servings

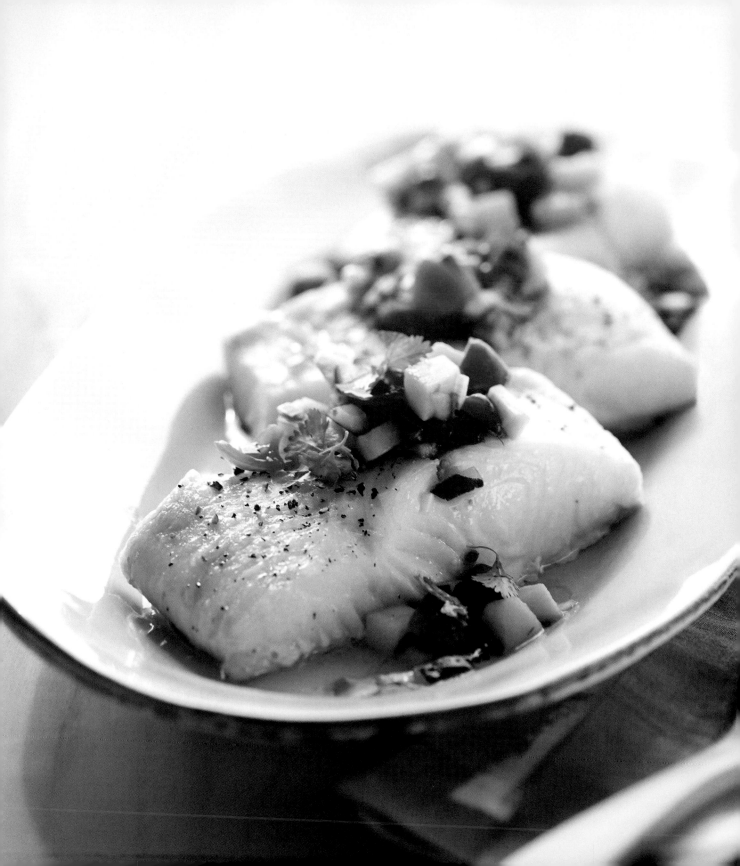

Halibut with Tomato-Mango Salsa

Halibut is a lean, mild, and sweet-tasting fish with a firm but tender texture. The secret is not to overcook it.

TOTAL TIME: 35 MINUTES

¾ cup uncooked quinoa

2 cups water

SALSA

1 tomato, chopped

½ cup chopped mango

½ cup finely chopped red onion

¼ cup chopped cilantro

2 tablespoons lime juice

Sea salt

Ground black pepper

FISH

4 halibut or cod fillets (1½ pounds total)

½ tablespoon extra-virgin olive oil

Sea salt

Ground black pepper

In a saucepan over medium-high heat, combine the quinoa and water and bring to a boil. Reduce the heat to low, cover, and cook for 15 minutes, or until the water is absorbed. Set aside, covered, to steam for 5 minutes. Fluff the quinoa with a fork and transfer to a medium bowl.

To make the salsa: In a mixing bowl, combine the tomato, mango, onion, cilantro, and lime juice. Season with salt and pepper to taste and set aside.

To make the fish: Preheat the broiler. Lightly brush the fish with the oil and season lightly with salt and pepper. Place the fish on a shallow broiler pan and broil for 5 to 7 minutes on each side, or until it flakes easily. (The thickness of the fish will determine the cooking time.)

Place each fillet on a plate and top with the salsa. Serve with the quinoa.

Makes 4 servings

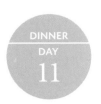

Fish Tacos with Mango-Avocado Salsa

Fish tacos served in restaurants are often battered and deep-fried. There's no need for that. Giving the fish a quick turn in the skillet allows its freshness to shine through. Some Mango-Avocado Salsa is a nice change-up from tomato salsa.

TOTAL TIME: 30 MINUTES

1 cup shredded cabbage

1 avocado, pitted, peeled, and chopped

1 mango, pitted, peeled, and chopped

2 tablespoons chopped red onion

2 tablespoons chopped cilantro

1 tablespoon lime juice

Sea salt

Ground black pepper

½ teaspoon extra-virgin olive oil

1 pound cod or mahi mahi fillets

8 corn tortillas (6" diameter), warmed

Lime wedges

In a medium bowl, combine the cabbage, avocado, mango, onion, cilantro, lime juice, and salt and pepper to taste. Set aside at room temperature.

In a large nonstick skillet over medium-high heat, heat the oil. Season the fillets lightly with salt and pepper and cook for 3 minutes on each side, or until the fish flakes easily. (The cooking time will depend on the thickness of the fish.)

Divide the fish and cabbage salad among the tortillas and serve with lime wedges.

Makes 4 servings

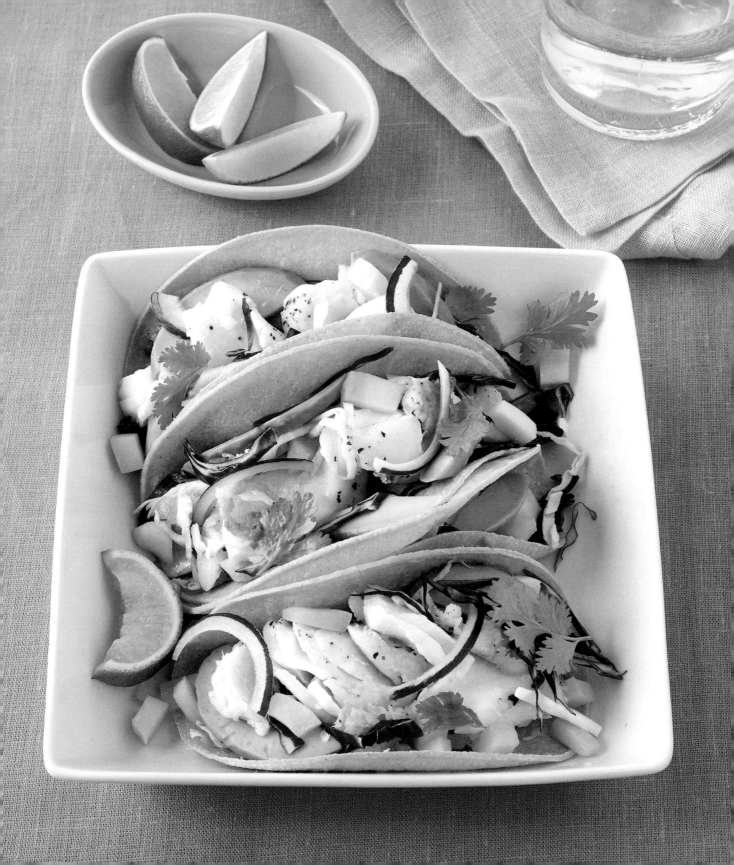

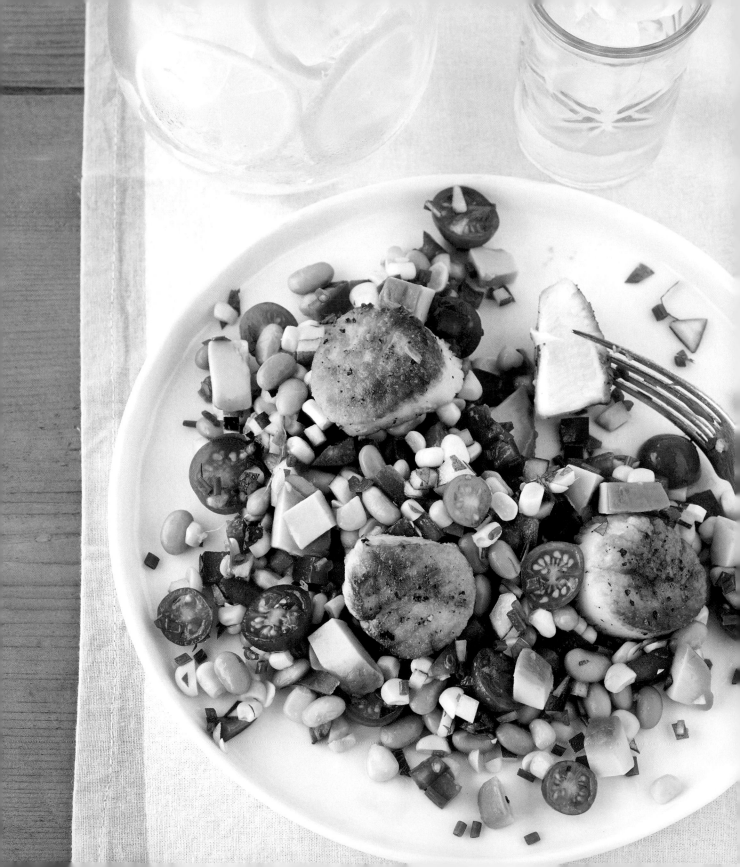

Seared Scallops and Succotash

DINNER
DAY
12

Grown in deep ocean waters, meaty sea scallops are 1 to 2 inches in diameter and are best when quickly seared or grilled. Dry the scallops thoroughly, so they become crispy in the pan. If using fresh corn, remove the kernels from 1 to 2 ears.

TOTAL TIME: 30 MINUTES

3 cups water

¾ cup fresh or frozen corn kernels

½ cup baby lima beans or edamame

1 cup quartered cherry tomatoes

1 avocado, pitted, peeled, and chopped

1 red bell pepper, chopped

½ cup chopped red onion

¼ cup chopped fresh flat-leaf parsley

4 tablespoons extra-virgin olive oil, divided

Juice of ½ lemon

1 clove garlic, chopped

Sea salt

1 pound sea scallops

Ground black pepper

2 tablespoons chopped fresh chives

In a medium saucepan, bring the water to a boil. Simmer the corn and lima beans or edamame for 3 minutes, or until tender. Drain. When cool, transfer to a large bowl and add the tomatoes, avocado, bell pepper, onion, and parsley.

In a small bowl, whisk together 2 tablespoons of the oil, the lemon juice, garlic, and ¼ teaspoon of salt. Drizzle the dressing over the vegetables and toss well. Taste and adjust the seasoning, if needed. Set aside.

Pat the scallops dry with paper towels and then season with salt and pepper. In a large skillet over medium-high heat, heat the remaining 2 tablespoons oil until shimmering. Place the scallops at least 1" apart in the skillet and cook undisturbed for 2 minutes, or until the bottom edges are golden and they release easily. Gently turn the scallops and cook for 1 to 2 minutes, or until opaque on the inside and golden brown on the outside.

Divide the succotash among 4 serving plates and top with the scallops. Sprinkle with the chives before serving.

Makes 4 servings

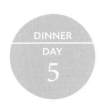

Flank Steak with Arugula

Lean flank steak has a nice beefy flavor, and it takes well to all kinds of marinades, like this one made with lime juice, garlic, and balsamic vinegar. Flank steak is best when grilled to rare or medium-rare, then sliced and layered on some peppery arugula.

TOTAL TIME: 30 MINUTES

Juice of 2 limes

2 cloves garlic, minced

3 tablespoons balsamic vinegar

1 teaspoon extra-virgin olive oil

¼ teaspoon sea salt

¼ teaspoon ground black pepper

1 pound flank steak

5 ounces arugula

¼ cup White Balsamic Vinaigrette (page 159)

In a resealable plastic bag, combine the lime juice, garlic, vinegar, oil, salt, and pepper. Add the steak and shake gently to coat. Put the sealed bag in a shallow dish and refrigerate for 10 to 15 minutes.

Preheat a grill pan over medium-high heat. Lift the steak from the bag and let any excess marinade drip off. Discard the marinade. Grill the steak for 5 to 7 minutes on each side for medium-rare or until a thermometer inserted in the center registers 145°F. Transfer the steak to a cutting board and let it rest for 5 to 10 minutes to reabsorb its juices. Thinly slice the steak across the grain.

In a medium bowl, toss the arugula with the vinaigrette. Divide the salad among 4 plates, top with the sliced steak, and serve.

Makes 4 servings

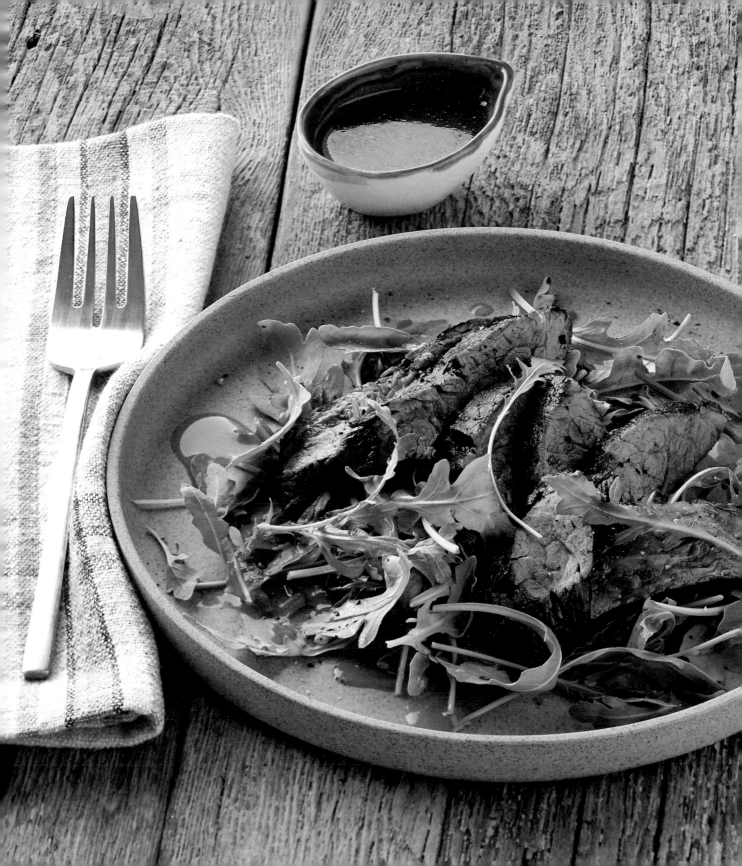

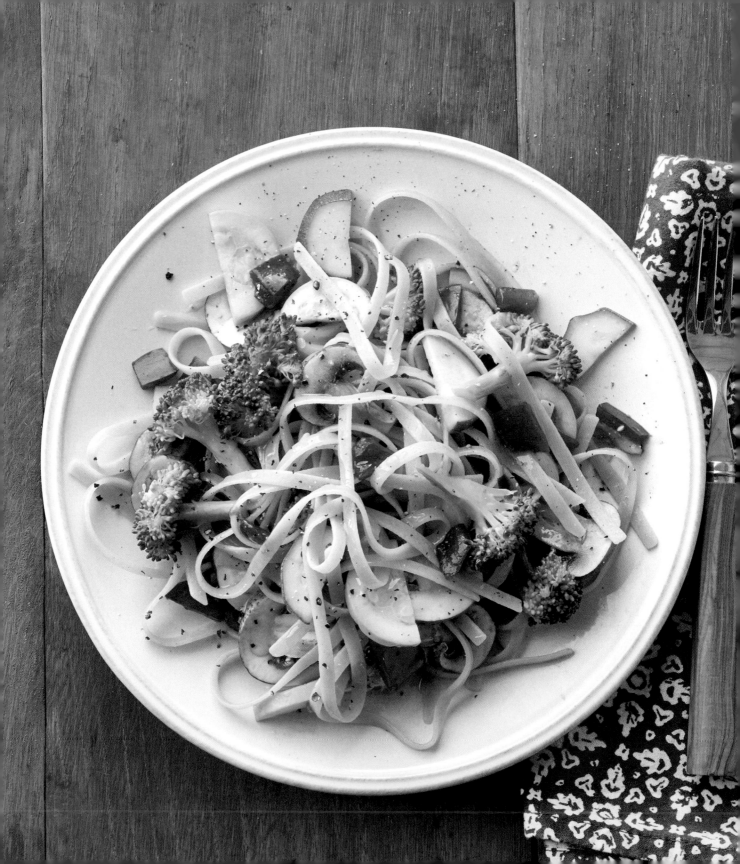

Pasta Primavera

DINNER
DAY
4

Primavera means spring in Italian. Even though the original preparation featured just spring-time vegetables—fresh peas, tiny asparagus, and small onions—pasta primavera is made with seasonal vegetables throughout the year. I like to include broccoli, mushrooms, and summer squash, but feel free to use cauliflower, carrots, and red or yellow bell peppers.

TOTAL TIME: 20 MINUTES

8 ounces brown rice fettuccine

1 cup broccoli florets

½ cup sliced mushrooms

½ cup sliced zucchini

½ cup sliced yellow squash

1 teaspoon extra-virgin olive oil

1 large tomato, chopped

1 clove garlic, minced (optional)

Sea salt

Ground black pepper

Prepare the pasta according to package directions.

In a large saucepan with a steamer basket, bring 1" of water to a boil. Steam the broccoli, mushrooms, zucchini, and yellow squash in the basket for 5 minutes, or until tender. (The time depends on the individual vegetables. The mushrooms will be tender before the squash, for instance.) Transfer to a colander to drain. Set aside.

In a large skillet over medium heat, heat the oil. Cook the tomato and garlic (if desired), stirring frequently, for 1 minute. Add the steamed vegetables, season with salt and pepper to taste, and cook for 1 minute. Place the pasta in a serving bowl and top with the vegetable mixture.

Makes 4 servings

Roasted Vegetable Pasta

It's no secret that pasta is one of America's favorite foods. With more than 600 shapes and sizes, there's something for everyone. This roasted vegetable pasta recipe is made with wheat-free brown rice pasta. We eat this dish almost weekly in my house. Feel free to substitute quinoa pasta.

TOTAL TIME: 30 MINUTES

8	ounces brown rice rotini pasta (or other preferred shape)
½	pint cherry tomatoes
8	cremini mushrooms, sliced
½	yellow onion, sliced
8–10	asparagus spears, trimmed and cut into 2" pieces
1	clove garlic, thinly sliced
2	tablespoons extra-virgin olive oil
½	teaspoon sea salt
¼	teaspoon ground black pepper
¼	cup chopped basil leaves
12	Parmesan shavings, each about 2" long (optional)

Cook the pasta according to package directions.

Preheat the oven to 450°F.

In a medium bowl, combine the tomatoes, mushrooms, onion, asparagus, and garlic. Add the oil, salt, and pepper and toss well to coat thoroughly. Arrange the vegetables in a single layer in a baking dish and bake for 10 minutes. Turn the vegetables over and cook for 10 minutes, or until they're tender and lightly browned. Remove from the oven. Divide the pasta and vegetables among 4 plates and top with the basil and Parmesan shavings (if desired).

Makes 4 servings

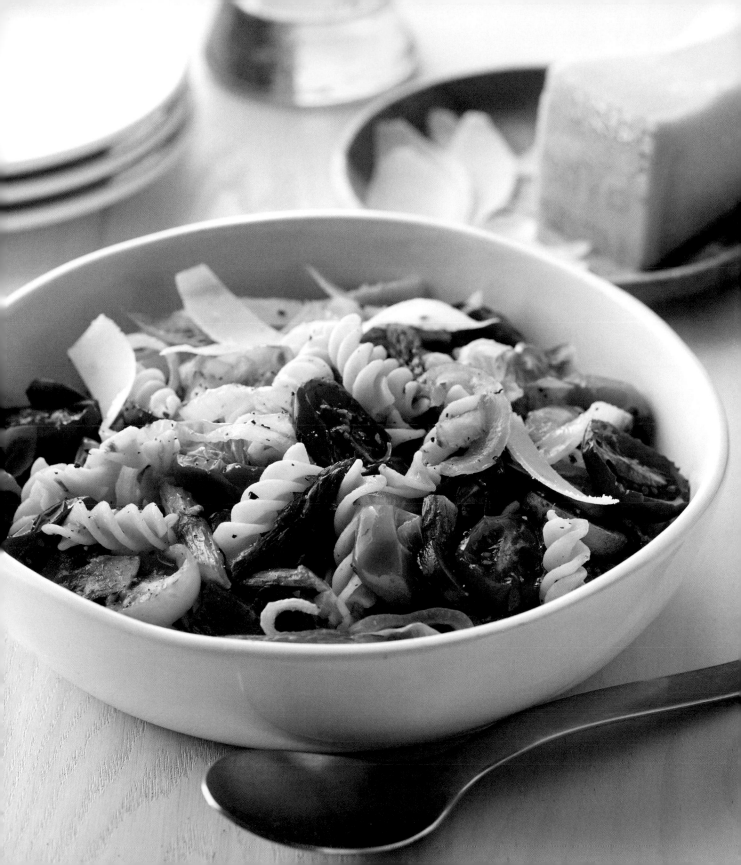

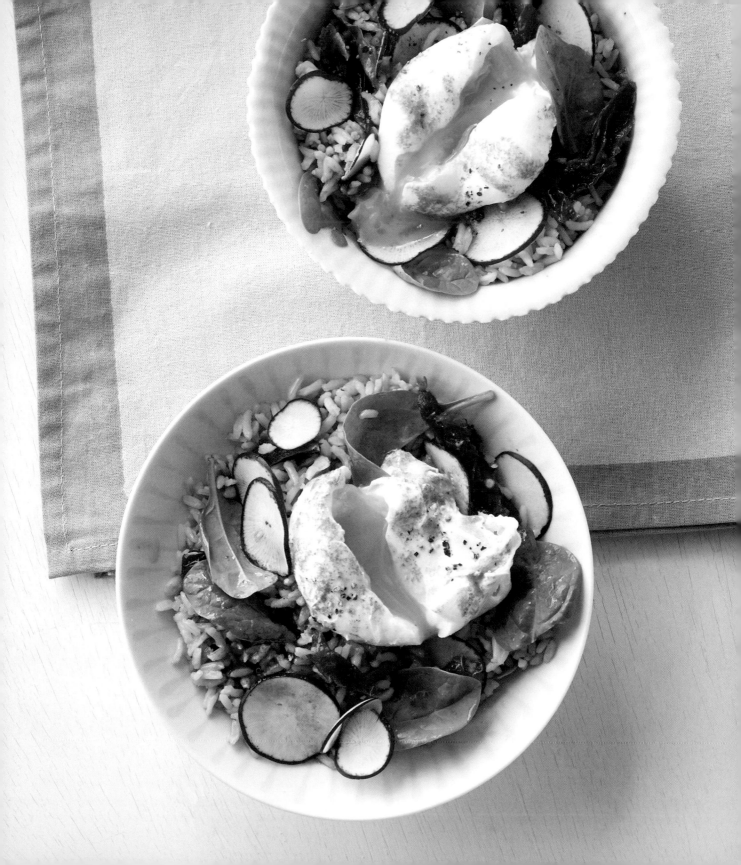

Poached Egg Rice Bowl with Basil Oil

This rice bowl is a take on bibimbap, the popular Korean dish of rice topped with an egg and vegetables. I like to drizzle on some bright green basil oil for a colorful touch.

TOTAL TIME: 45 MINUTES

1 cup uncooked long-grain brown rice

2¼ cups + 2 tablespoons water

Sea salt

½ cup packed fresh basil leaves

¼ cup extra-virgin olive oil

2 tablespoons distilled vinegar or rice vinegar

4 large eggs

3 cups baby spinach or baby kale leaves

⅔ cup thinly sliced radishes

½ cup sliced, dry-packed sun-dried tomatoes

Ground black pepper

In a medium saucepan, combine the rice and 2¼ cups of the water. Add a pinch of salt and bring to a boil over medium-high heat. Reduce the heat to low, cover, and simmer for 30 minutes, or until tender. Remove the pan from the heat and let stand, covered, for 10 minutes.

In a blender, combine the basil, oil, a pinch of salt, and the remaining 2 tablespoons water. Blend until almost smooth. Scrape down the sides of the blender's canister as needed. Add a little more water if needed to help with the blending. Strain through a fine-mesh sieve set over a bowl and press down with a spatula to extract as much oil as possible. Discard the solids.

Fill a large skillet with water. Add the vinegar and bring the water to a boil over high heat. Break the eggs into 4 separate teacups or small bowls. When the water comes to a boil, slide the pan off the heat and gently tip the eggs into the pan. Cover the pan tightly and let it sit for 4 minutes, or until the whites are set and the yolks are still runny.

Fluff the rice with a fork. Divide the rice among 4 serving bowls and top with the spinach or kale, radishes, and tomatoes. Using a slotted spoon, carefully remove the poached eggs from the water, letting the excess water drip off. Set 1 egg in each bowl, drizzle the basil oil over the eggs, and season to taste with black pepper.

Makes 4 servings

Mediterranean Flatbread Pizzas

Those who know me well know that flatbread pizza is one of my favorite indulgences. The flatbreads and pesto can be made up to 3 days in advance, but assemble the pizzas just before cooking them. The pesto recipe makes more than you'll need for these pizzas; keep leftover pesto to use on wraps or as a pasta topping.

TOTAL TIME: 1 HOUR 30 MINUTES

FLATBREADS

1 large egg

¾ cup brown rice flour

½ cup quinoa flour

1 tablespoon chopped fresh rosemary or thyme

¼ teaspoon sea salt

1 cup water

PESTO

1 cup cilantro

1 cup fresh basil leaves

⅓ cup grated Parmesan cheese

¼ cup walnut pieces

2 cloves garlic, chopped

Juice of ½ lemon

¼ cup extra-virgin olive oil

TOPPINGS

1 tablespoon extra-virgin olive oil

½ cup drained and sliced marinated artichoke hearts

1 cup quartered cherry tomatoes

⅓ cup pitted and sliced kalamata olives

3 ounces soft goat cheese, crumbled

2 tablespoons capers, drained (optional)

To make the flatbreads: In a large bowl, lightly beat the egg. Stir in the rice flour, quinoa flour, rosemary or thyme, and salt. While stirring, slowly add the water and gently mix. The batter should be the consistency of pancake batter. If too thick, stir in more water a tablespoon at a time. If too runny, stir in additional flour a tablespoon at a time. Let the dough sit at room temperature for 1 hour, or until double in bulk.

To make the pesto: In a food processor, combine the cilantro, basil, Parmesan, walnuts, garlic, and lemon juice. Pulse until coarsely minced. With the machine running, pour the oil through the feed tube in a slow stream until the pesto is smooth. Pour the pesto into a bowl, cover, and set aside.

Heat an 8" or 10" cast-iron or nonstick skillet over medium heat. Pour ½ cup of the batter into the pan and rotate it in a circular motion to spread the batter over the bottom of the pan. Cook for 2 to 3 minutes, or until the underside of the flatbread browns. Turn and cook for 2 minutes, or until golden on both sides. Repeat with the remaining batter to make 4 flatbreads.

Preheat the oven to 350°F. Put the breads on a baking sheet (you may need 2 baking sheets) and spread 2 to 3 tablespoons of the reserved pesto on top of each. Top each with equal amounts of oil, artichoke hearts, tomatoes, olives, goat cheese, and capers (if desired). Bake for 8 to 10 minutes, or until the toppings and flatbreads are warmed through and the cheese melts.

Makes 4 servings

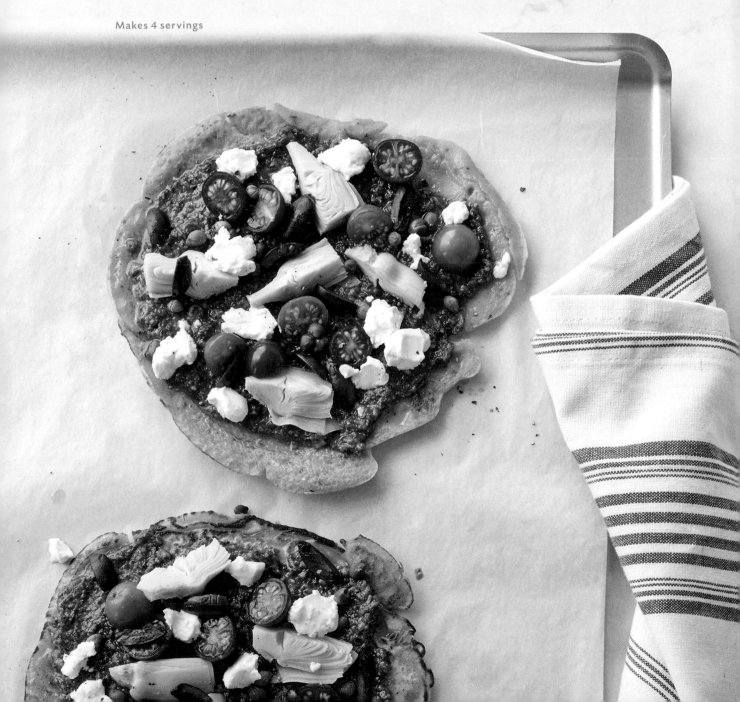

Shrimp and Broccoli Stir-Fry

When stir-frying, it's important to prep all of the ingredients and have them organized near the stove. This way, you can easily and efficiently add them to the pan when things start happening quickly. Broccoli florets are a great addition to this stir-fry, which is given a little heat from the sambal oelek, or chile paste. This stir-fry packs a protein punch by using quinoa instead of rice.

TOTAL TIME: 30 MINUTES

2 cups water

1 cup quinoa

½ cup orange juice

2 tablespoons gluten-free, reduced-sodium soy sauce or tamari

1 tablespoon minced fresh ginger

2 teaspoons toasted sesame oil

2 teaspoons sambal oelek

2 teaspoons cornstarch

¼ teaspoon ground black pepper

1 tablespoon peanut oil

1 pound large shrimp, peeled and deveined

1 large red bell pepper, thinly sliced

1 head broccoli, cut into florets

2 cups chopped pineapple

½ cup unsalted roasted cashews

3 scallions, thinly sliced

In a saucepan over medium-high heat, combine the quinoa and water and bring to a boil. Reduce the heat to low, cover, and cook for 15 minutes, or until the water is absorbed. Set aside, covered, to steam for 5 minutes. Fluff the quinoa with a fork and transfer to a medium bowl.

In a medium bowl, whisk together the orange juice, soy sauce or tamari, ginger, sesame oil, sambal oelek, cornstarch, and black pepper and set aside.

Heat a wok or large skillet over medium-high heat. Add the peanut oil, swirl to coat, and cook the shrimp for 2 minutes, or just until opaque. Remove the shrimp from the pan and set aside. Add the bell pepper and broccoli to the wok and cook, stirring constantly, for 3 minutes, or just until the vegetables are tender-crisp. Return the reserved shrimp to the wok along with the pineapple, cashews, and scallions. Pour in the reserved orange sauce, toss to coat, and heat for 1 minute.

Divide the quinoa among 4 plates and top with the shrimp stir-fry. Spoon any remaining orange sauce over the shrimp.

Makes 4 servings

Crab Cakes

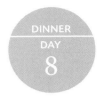

Crab cakes are a treat anytime, but they are especially welcome on the first day of the Clean Phase of the Healthy You Diet. My crab cakes are flavorful and light, but still filling. Serve them with a side of steamed green beans (page 212).

TOTAL TIME: 20 MINUTES

1 pound lump crab, cleaned of shell pieces

2 large egg whites

2 shallots, finely chopped

¼ cup finely chopped green or red bell pepper

¼ cup unsweetened almond milk

2 tablespoons Dijon mustard

2 tablespoons finely chopped fresh Italian parsley

1 teaspoon crab-boil seasoning

1 teaspoon ground white pepper

2 tablespoons gluten-free oat flour

1 tablespoon extra-virgin olive oil

Lemon wedges

In a medium bowl, combine the crab, egg whites, shallots, bell pepper, almond milk, mustard, parsley, crab-boil seasoning, and white pepper just until mixed. Divide into 8 small cakes. In a shallow dish, place the oat flour. Lightly coat each crab cake on both sides with the oat flour.

In a large skillet over medium heat, heat the oil and swirl to coat the pan. Cook the crab cakes for 8 to 12 minutes, turning once, or until golden. Serve with lemon wedges.

Makes 4 servings

Penne and Pesto

While pesto can be served on any pasta, I use penne or another short shape like fusilli. Make the pesto ahead or prepare it while the pasta is cooking. Some people like a smooth, creamy puree, while others prefer a little coarseness so they can taste the nuts. It's up to you. Stir the pesto into the hot pasta just before serving.

TOTAL TIME: 15 MINUTES

¼ cup toasted pine nuts or walnuts (see page 63)

2 cups fresh basil leaves

1 clove garlic

¼ teaspoon sea salt

¼ teaspoon ground black pepper

¼ cup extra-virgin olive oil

12 ounces brown rice pasta (such as penne or fusilli)

In a food processor, pulse the nuts until finely ground. Add the basil, garlic, salt, and pepper and pulse until finely chopped. With the food processor running, add the oil in a slow stream until the pesto reaches the desired consistency.

Prepare the pasta according to package directions. Divide the pasta among 4 bowls and top each with some of the pesto.

Makes 4 servings

Black Bean Tostadas with Salsa

Spicy black beans are great on toasted tortillas, topped with homemade salsa. Toasting the tortillas in the oven makes them crispy and aromatic. This is one of my go-to meals on busy weeknights when I don't have a lot of time to pull dinner together.

TOTAL TIME: 20 MINUTES

SALSA

- ½ cup chopped tomatoes
- ½ avocado, peeled and chopped
- 1 tablespoon finely chopped onion
- 1 tablespoon minced jalapeño chile pepper (optional; wear plastic gloves when handling)
- ⅛ teaspoon sea salt
- 2 teaspoons lime juice

BLACK BEANS

- 2 cans (15 ounces each) black beans, rinsed and drained
- ¼ cup hot sauce
- 2 tablespoons water

- 8 corn tortillas (6" diameter)
- 1 cup shredded lettuce

Preheat the oven to 350°F.

To make the salsa: In a small bowl, combine the tomatoes, avocado, onion, pepper (if desired), salt, and lime juice.

To make the beans: In a blender or food processor, combine the beans, hot sauce, and water. Blend or process until smooth. Pour the bean mixture into a saucepan and heat over low heat.

Arrange the tortillas on a baking sheet or place them directly on the oven rack and bake for 6 to 10 minutes, turning once, or until they become crispy and start to brown.

Top each tortilla with some of the warmed black beans, salsa, and lettuce before serving.

Makes 4 servings

chapter

15

appetizers and side dishes

I often bring some of the dishes in this chapter to family gatherings and parties. A bowl of White Bean Dip (page 199) surrounded with colorful vegetables or some fresh guacamole and homemade tortilla chips ensure there will be something healthy and delicious to nibble on. A platter of Roasted Brussels Sprouts and Carrots (page 211) is always welcome at holiday time.

White Bean Dip

Surround a bowl of this white bean dip with a rainbow of carrots, endive leaves, radishes, bell pepper strips, cucumbers, snow peas, blanched green beans, and broccoli and cauliflower florets. Vegetables never looked—or tasted—so good. Double or triple the recipe for a party.

TOTAL TIME: 15 MINUTES

    1 can (15 ounces) cannellini or great Northern beans, rinsed and drained
    1 clove garlic, minced
    ½ yellow onion, thinly sliced
    2 tablespoons extra-virgin olive oil
    1 tablespoon lemon juice
    1 tablespoon finely chopped fresh parsley
    ½ teaspoon sea salt
    ¼ teaspoon ground black pepper
    1 tablespoon water (optional)

In a food processor, combine the beans, garlic, onion, oil, lemon juice, parsley, salt, and pepper. Pulse until smooth. If the dip is too thick, add the water and pulse to mix. Serve with vegetables of your choosing.

Makes 4 servings (1¼ to 1½ cups)

Guacamole

I'm a huge fan of guacamole—it's healthy and light, and it brightens up so many dishes. I add a spoonful to bean soups or chilis or use it to top off my chicken and seafood tacos, crab cakes, or scrambled eggs. If you ask me, everything tastes better with a dollop of guac!

TOTAL TIME: 10 MINUTES

2 avocados, pitted and flesh scooped out

2 tablespoons Fresh Salsa (page 204)

¼ medium red onion, chopped

1 tablespoon chopped cilantro

1½ teaspoons fresh lime juice

1 teaspoon sea salt

½ teaspoon minced garlic

½ teaspoon ground cumin

¼ teaspoon chili powder

Corn tortilla or flax chips

In a large bowl, combine the avocados, salsa, onion, cilantro, lime juice, salt, garlic, cumin, and chili powder. Mash with a fork or potato masher to desired consistency. Serve immediately with the chips, or cover and refrigerate for 1 hour before serving.

Makes 3 servings (approximately 1½ cups)

Hummus with Vegetables

Although a new brand of hummus seems to be introduced to the market every day, I still prefer to make my own unprocessed version at home. I usually double the recipe so there is always some hummus ready to snack on with a handful of fresh vegetables.

TOTAL TIME: 10 MINUTES

1 clove garlic, crushed

2 tablespoons tahini

2 tablespoons fresh lime juice

1 tablespoon extra-virgin olive oil

¾ teaspoon sea salt

1 can (15 ounces) chickpeas, rinsed and drained

1–2 tablespoons water (optional)

Carrot and celery sticks, sliced bell peppers, sliced cucumbers, romaine lettuce leaves, and other vegetables of your choosing

In a food processor, combine the garlic, tahini, lime juice, oil, and salt. Process for 30 seconds. Scrape the mixture from the sides of the food processor. Add half of the chickpeas and process for 1 minute. Scrape the mixture from the sides and add the remaining chickpeas. If you prefer a thinner consistency, add the water as needed and blend well. Transfer the hummus to a bowl and serve with fresh vegetables. Cover and refrigerate any leftover hummus for up to 3 days.

Makes 3 servings (approximately 1½ cups)

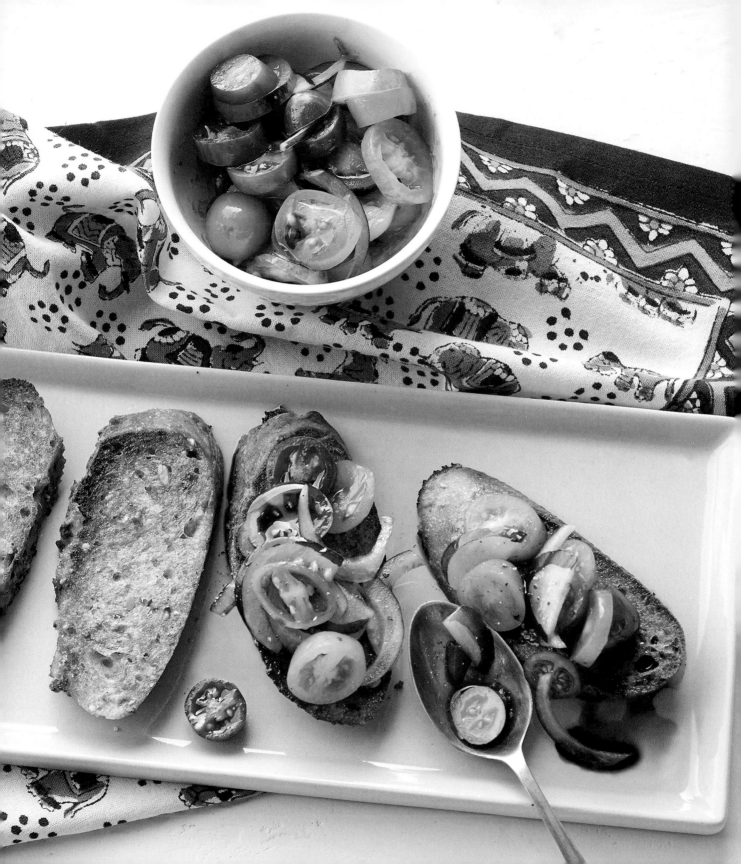

Cherry Tomato Bruschetta

When making bruschetta, an Italian antipasto of grilled bread topped with tomatoes, I like to use a variety of cherry tomatoes. Cherry tomatoes come in a rainbow of colors—from bright yellow to deep gold, from pale pink to fire engine red, from lime to avocado green.

TOTAL TIME: 45 MINUTES

1 pint cherry tomatoes, halved

¼ red onion, thinly sliced

2 tablespoons extra-virgin olive oil, divided

1 tablespoon balsamic vinegar

¼ teaspoon sea salt

⅛ teaspoon ground black pepper

8 wheat-free baguette slices (½" thick) or 4 slices wheat-free bread

Preheat the broiler.

In a medium bowl, combine the tomatoes, onion, 1 tablespoon of the oil, vinegar, salt, and pepper. Toss well. Set aside at room temperature for 30 minutes.

Arrange the bread slices on a baking sheet. Brush the slices with the remaining 1 tablespoon oil. Broil for 1 to 2 minutes, or just until toasted on 1 side. Watch carefully, as the bread can burn quickly.

Divide the tomato mixture among the toasts and serve.

Makes 4 servings

SNACK

DAY

8

Fresh Salsa and Tortilla Chips

I *love* chips and salsa! It's something I didn't want to give up while trying to lose weight. Instead of writing it off, I figured out how to make a healthier version. It may not be as convenient as opening a bag of chips and a jar of salsa, but making your own is worth the extra effort.

TOTAL TIME: 15 MINUTES

SALSA

3 tomatoes, chopped

½ cup finely chopped onion

1 small jalapeño chile pepper, seeded and minced (optional; wear plastic gloves when handling)

¼ cup minced cilantro

2 tablespoons lime juice

Sea salt

TORTILLA CHIPS

8 100% corn tortillas

Sea salt

To make the salsa: In a mixing bowl, combine the tomatoes, onion, pepper, cilantro, and lime juice. Season to taste with salt.

To make the tortilla chips: Preheat the oven to 350°F.

Cut each tortilla into 4 to 6 triangular pieces. Arrange the pieces on a baking sheet and sprinkle lightly with salt. Bake for 10 to 12 minutes, flipping once, or until the pieces are crisp and just beginning to brown slightly. Remove the baking sheet from the oven and let the tortilla chips cool. Serve the chips with the salsa.

Makes 4 servings

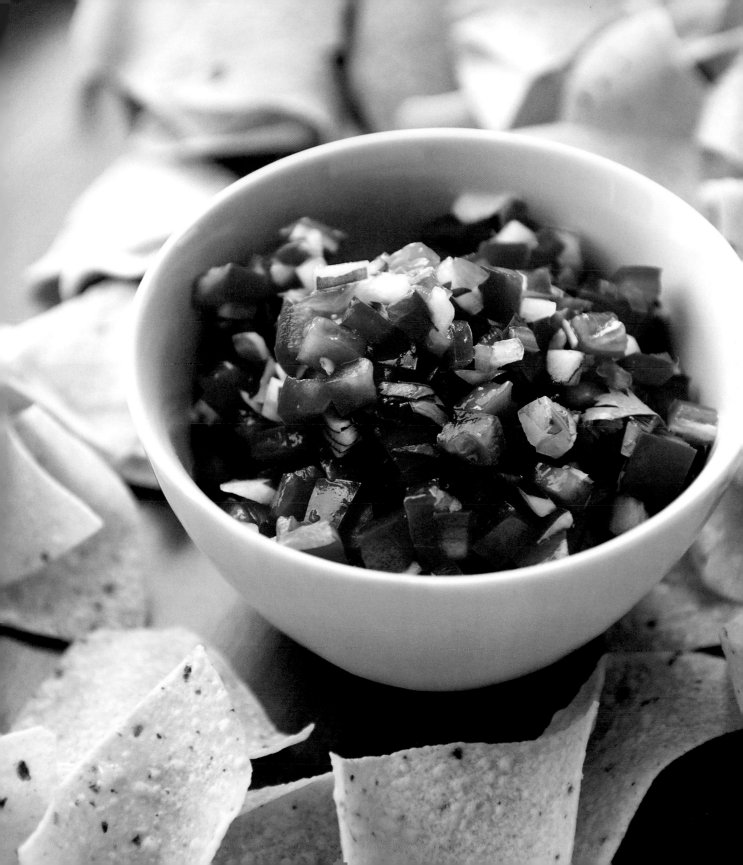

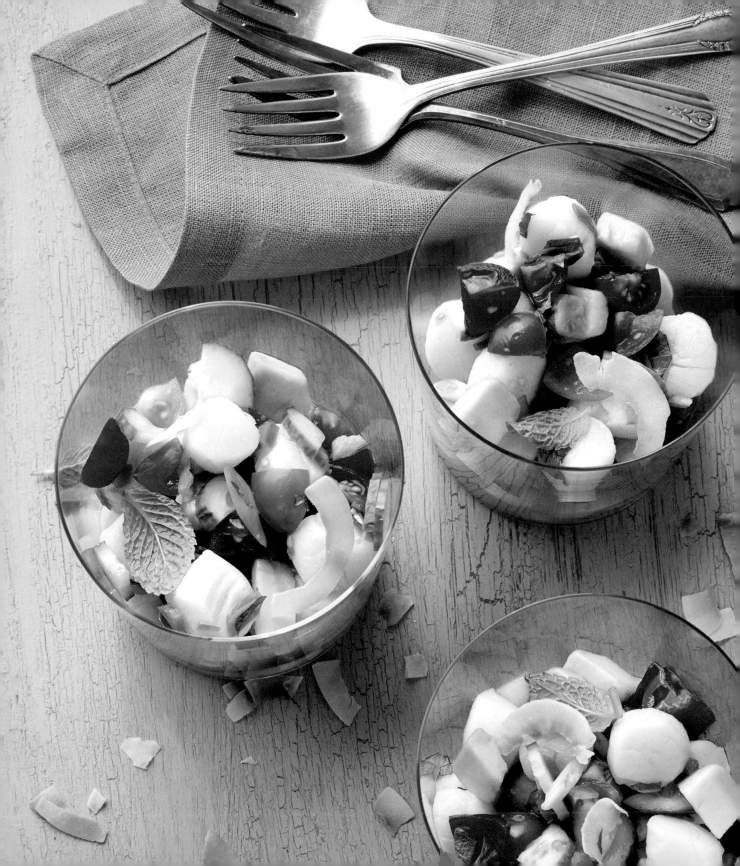

Scallop Ceviche

For this recipe, you want to purchase small bay scallops that come from shallow waters, not the larger sea scallops. Bay scallops are about ½ inch in size, making them just right for a bite of this citrusy ceviche. Enjoy this dish for lunch or serve it as a first course at a Mexican-themed dinner party.

TOTAL TIME: 15 MINUTES + CHILLING TIME

⅓ **cup fresh lemon juice**

⅓ **cup fresh lime juice, plus a little extra for serving**

⅓ **cup fresh orange juice**

1 **pound bay scallops**

1 **cup quartered cherry tomatoes**

1 **small avocado, pitted, peeled, and chopped**

½ **English cucumber, chopped**

2 **scallions, thinly sliced**

1 **clove garlic, minced**

⅓ **cup chopped mint leaves**

1 **serrano chile pepper or jalapeño chile pepper, seeded and minced
(wear plastic gloves when handling)**

¼ **cup dried unsweetened coconut flakes**

¼ **teaspoon sea salt**

In a nonreactive bowl, stir together the lemon juice, lime juice, and orange juice. Add the scallops, cover, and refrigerate for at least 3 hours or up to 8 hours. Stir the scallops once or twice during chilling.

When ready to serve, drain the scallops. Add the tomatoes, avocado, cucumber, scallions, garlic, mint, pepper, coconut, and salt and toss gently. Squeeze on some additional lime juice. Divide the ceviche among 4 or 8 serving glasses.

Makes 4 servings (main dish)

Makes 8 servings (appetizer)

Mango, Avocado, and Tomato Salad

This is a bright all-fruit salad—the tomato is botanically a fruit—that goes with grilled fish and seafood, chicken, and steak. I often make a huge bowl of it to bring to barbecues.

TOTAL TIME: 15 MINUTES

2 tablespoons fresh lime juice

1 tablespoon extra-virgin olive oil

1 tablespoon balsamic vinegar

¼ teaspoon sea salt

¼ teaspoon ground black pepper

1 mango, pitted, peeled, and sliced

1 avocado, pitted, peeled, and sliced

1 small tomato, sliced

1 tablespoon flat-leaf parsley leaves

In a small bowl, whisk together the lime juice, oil, vinegar, salt, and pepper. Set aside.

In a medium bowl, combine the mango, avocado, and tomato. Pour the dressing over the fruit, add the parsley, and toss to combine. Divide the salad between 2 plates and serve.

Makes 2 servings

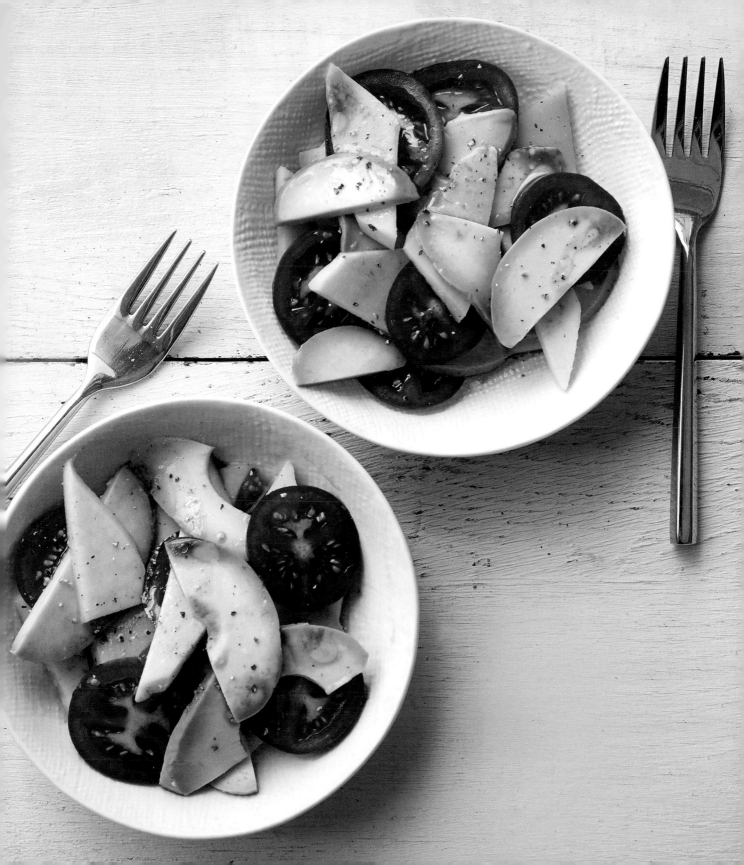

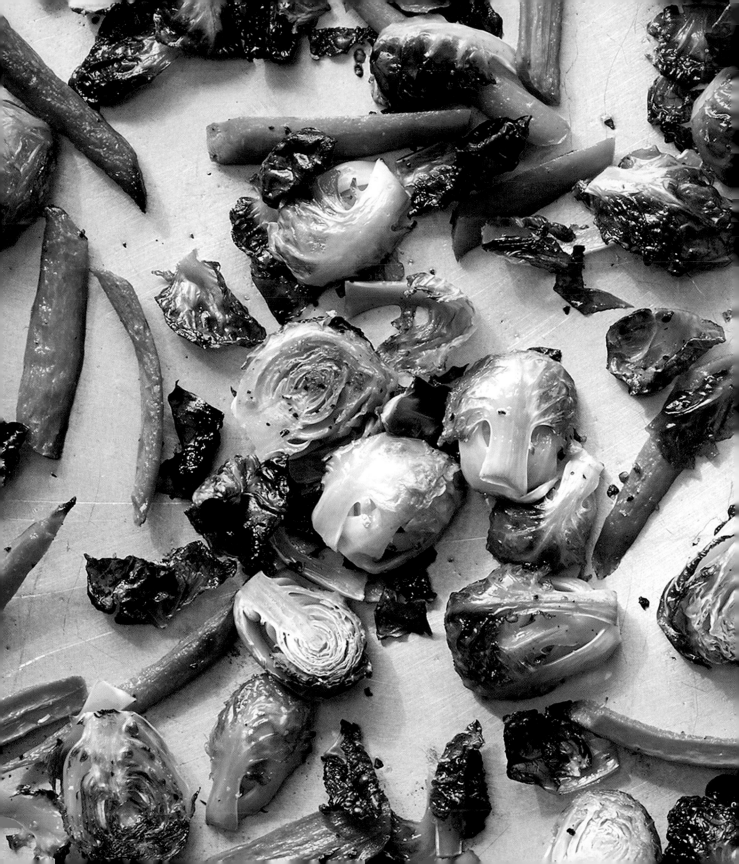

Roasted Brussels Sprouts and Carrots

VG WF GF DF

Roasting vegetables brings out their inherent sweetness. Try this method with summer squash, eggplant, peppers, onions, broccoli, cauliflower, fennel, and just about any vegetable you can think of. The amount of time required to make the vegetables soft on the inside, crisp outside will vary depending on how large the pieces are and which vegetables you use.

TOTAL TIME: 25 MINUTES

1 pound Brussels sprouts, trimmed and halved lengthwise

½ pound carrots, cut into 2" pieces

2 tablespoons extra-virgin olive oil

1 teaspoon sea salt

Preheat the oven to 425°F. In a medium bowl, combine the Brussels sprouts and carrots. Add the oil and salt and toss thoroughly to coat. Arrange the vegetables in a baking dish and roast for 20 minutes, turning once, or until the vegetables are tender and lightly browned.

Makes 4 servings

Steaming Vegetables

Looking for the perfect side dish that won't get in the way of your weight-loss goals? Steamed vegetables are always a healthy addition to any of the main meals. Feel free to steam and enjoy some green beans, asparagus, broccoli, and other vegetables.

Cooking vegetables over steaming (as opposed to in boiling) water helps them retain their color, texture, and vitamins. It is an easy procedure, but it works best if you have a good steaming setup. A collapsible stainless steel (or silicone) steamer is convenient because it folds away for storage, but a dedicated steamer/saucepan set is sturdier.

Here are the basic instructions for steaming vegetables on the stove with a collapsible steamer. First, choose a wide saucepan with a tight-fitting lid. Place the steamer in the saucepan and add enough cold water (no need to salt the water) to almost come up to the bottom of the steamer. Cover the saucepan and bring the water to a rolling boil over high heat to create a head of steam.

While the water is coming to a boil, prepare the vegetables, which should be cut into uniform pieces. Elongated vegetables like carrots and summer squash should be cut into rounds about ½ inch thick. Cruciferous broccoli and cauliflower can be cut into florets about 1 inch square. Green beans should be trimmed and cut into 1-inch lengths.

Add the vegetables to the steamer (watch out for escaping steam!). You don't have to season the vegetables at this point. Cover the saucepan tightly again and lower the heat so the water simmers at a good clip to maintain the steam. Now just steam the vegetables until they are done to your liking; I prefer tender-crisp, just firm enough that the tip of a knife can be inserted into the vegetable with a little pressure. Of course, the timing changes with each vegetable, but start testing after the 5-minute mark. Try not to test too often because you'll allow the built-up steam to escape. Using a pot holder, grab the central stem and remove the steamer. Transfer the vegetables to a serving dish, add your seasonings, and serve.

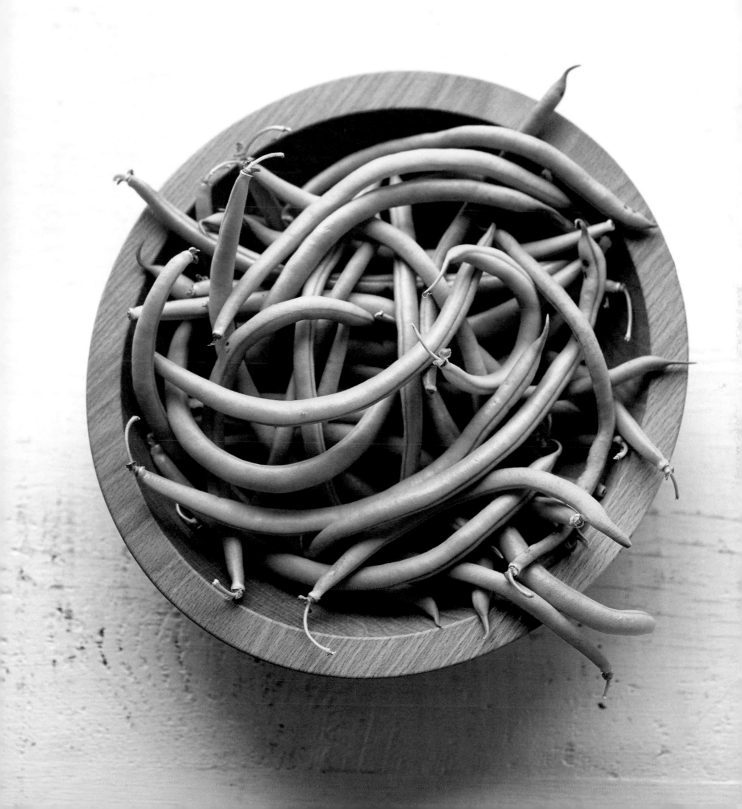

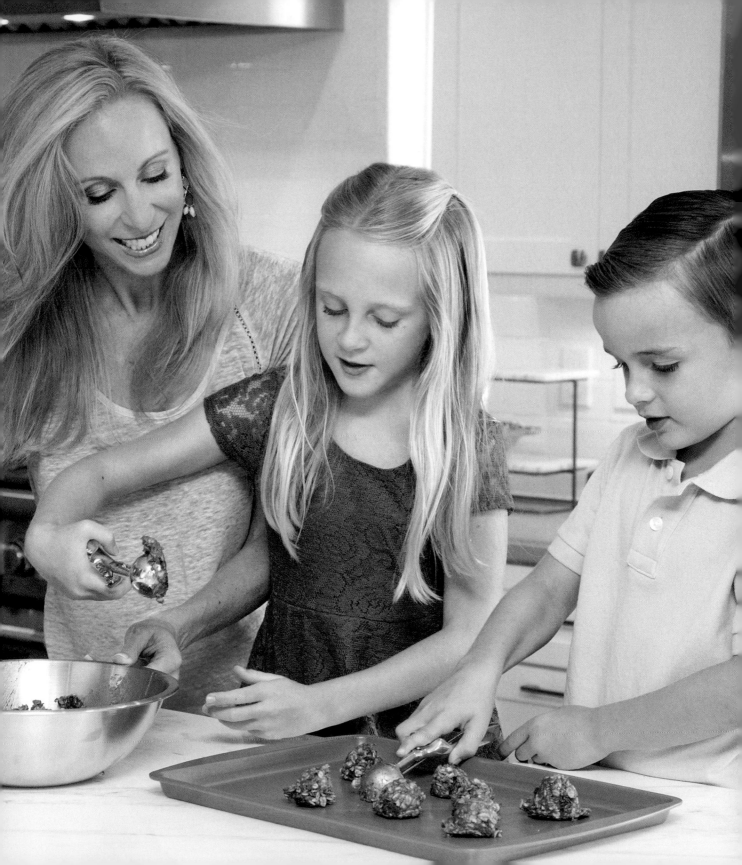

chapter

desserts and snacks

I'm a huge fan of desserts. People often wonder how I can eat cookies, cakes, pies, and ice cream and still stay fit, thin, and healthy. Life wouldn't be any fun without dessert—especially chocolate—but moderation is the key. I eat clean 80 to 90 percent of the time so that when I do indulge in dessert, I don't feel guilty about it. The desserts in this chapter are all free of wheat, gluten, and dairy. Most are also free from highly refined sugar. When you want something sweet, you'll find satisfaction here.

Chocolate Chip–Banana Cake

For me, this chocolate-banana combination is as close to a perfect dessert as I can get. The bananas add luscious moistness, and the chocolate chips provide a welcome sweet wallop.

TOTAL TIME: 45 MINUTES

2 cups gluten-free oat flour

1½ teaspoons gluten-free baking powder

½ teaspoon baking soda

½ teaspoon sea salt

¼ teaspoon ground nutmeg

1 cup mashed ripe bananas (2–3 bananas)

2 large eggs

¼ cup honey

¼ cup unsweetened almond milk

3 tablespoons melted coconut oil

1 teaspoon vanilla extract

½ cup gluten-free dark chocolate chips

Preheat the oven to 350°F. Lightly oil an 8" × 8" baking pan.

In a large bowl, whisk together the flour, baking powder, baking soda, salt, and nutmeg.

In a mixing bowl, combine the bananas, eggs, honey, almond milk, oil, and vanilla and beat with a fork. Pour into the dry ingredients and mix well. Gently mix in the chocolate chips. Pour the batter into the pan. Bake for 25 to 30 minutes, or until a wooden pick inserted in the center comes out clean. Cool in the pan on a rack.

Makes 9 servings

Flourless Chocolate Cake

Every chocolate lover on the planet will appreciate a slice of this rich, yummy flourless chocolate cake. I'm no exception. This sinfully and satisfyingly chocolaty cake is made with almond milk, coconut oil, and a good amount of dark chocolate.

TOTAL TIME: 1 HOUR + CHILLING TIME

½ cup melted coconut oil

½ cup unsweetened almond milk

5 large eggs

2 bars (4 ounces each) gluten-free dark chocolate, broken into pieces

1½ teaspoons vanilla extract

¼ cup unsweetened cocoa powder

Preheat the oven to 350°F. Lightly oil a 9" springform pan with a little of the coconut oil. Line the bottom of the pan with parchment paper.

In a small saucepan over medium-high heat, heat the milk to a simmer and then remove from the heat. (Alternately, this can be done in the microwave.)

Into a blender, break the eggs and blend on medium speed for 1 minute, or until they are light lemon in color. Transfer to a bowl and set aside. Put the chocolate pieces in the blender and add the remaining oil and the hot milk. Cover the blender and let the mixture stand for 2 minutes. Blend on medium speed until smooth. Add the vanilla, cocoa, and reserved eggs and blend on medium speed until well mixed, scraping down the sides of the blender a few times.

Pour the batter into the pan and bake for 20 to 25 minutes, or until a wooden pick inserted 2" from the center of the cake comes out clean. Cool in the pan on a rack. When cool, refrigerate the cake for 2 to 3 hours. To serve, release and remove the sides of the springform pan.

Makes 12 servings

Rustic Cranberry Cake

It's easy to be tempted by unhealthy desserts during the holiday season. Make this simple cake and put it on your dessert table. By opting for frozen cranberries, you can make this any time of the year.

TOTAL TIME: 1 HOUR 15 MINUTES

½ cup gluten-free oat flour

½ cup almond flour

5 tablespoons coconut palm sugar, divided

1 tablespoon coconut flour

¼ teaspoon sea salt

2 cups fresh or frozen cranberries (thawed and drained, if using frozen)

½ cup chopped walnuts, divided

2 large eggs

½ cup fresh orange juice

¼ cup melted coconut oil

¼ cup honey

1 teaspoon almond extract

Preheat the oven to 350°F. Lightly oil a 9" pie plate.

In a large bowl, combine the oat flour, almond flour, 4 tablespoons of the sugar, coconut flour, and salt. Stir in the cranberries and ¼ cup of the walnuts. Toss to coat the berries and nuts with the flour mixture.

In a mixing bowl, beat the eggs. Add the orange juice, oil, honey, and almond extract and whisk until well mixed. Add to the dry ingredients and mix well. (The batter will be thick if using frozen berries.) Spread the batter into the pie plate and sprinkle with the remaining ¼ cup walnuts and 1 tablespoon sugar. Bake for 35 to 45 minutes, or until a wooden pick inserted in the center of the cake comes out clean. Serve warm or at room temperature.

Makes 8 servings

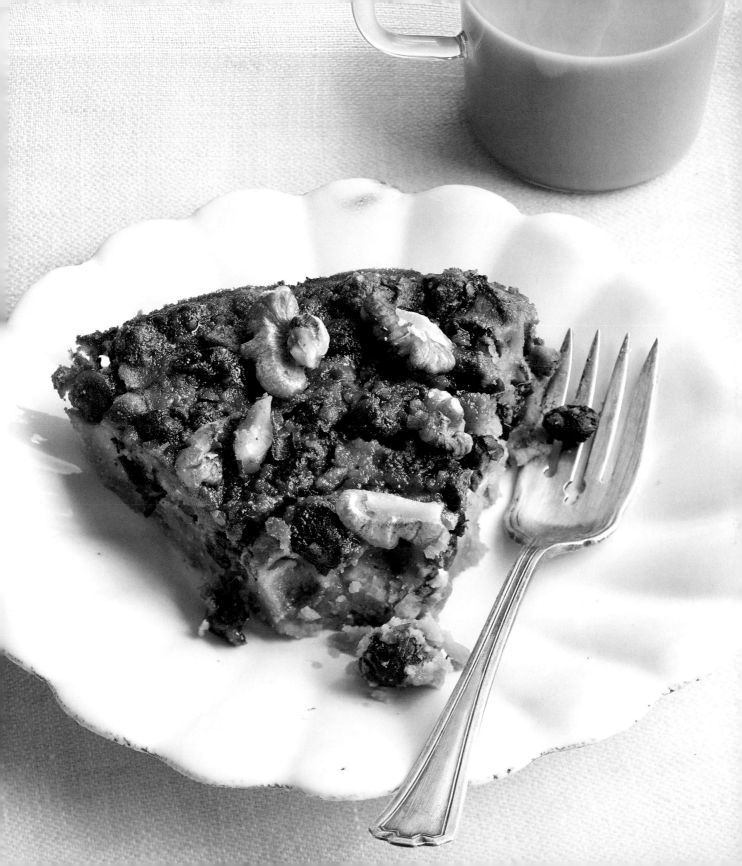

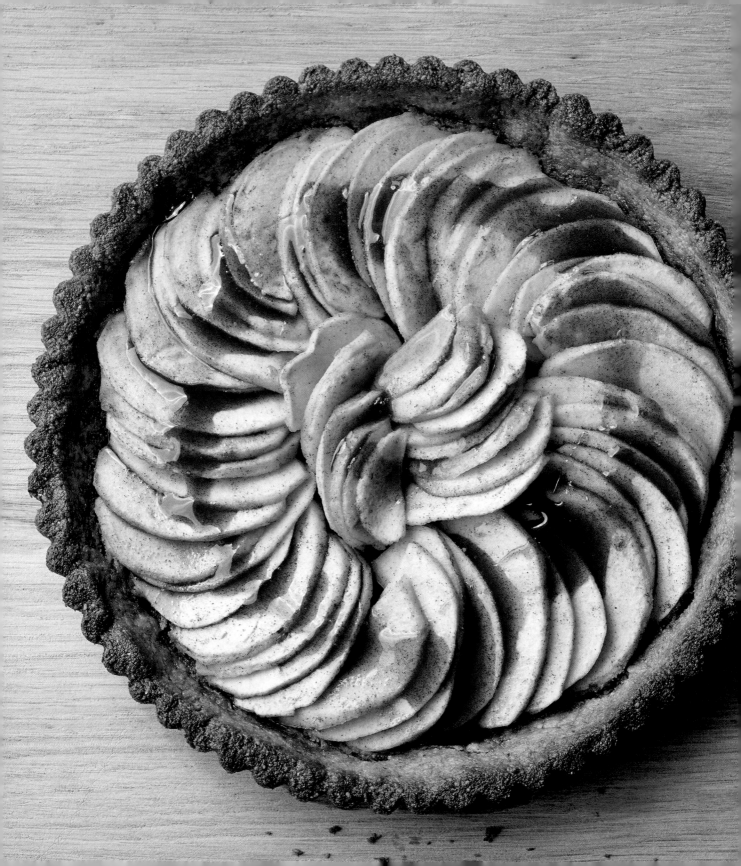

Apple-Walnut Tart

Yes, you can bake desserts without refined sugar! Maple syrup and orange juice are used to sweeten the apple filling. Try this tart when new-crop apples can be found at farmers' markets in the autumn.

TOTAL TIME: 1 HOUR 30 MINUTES

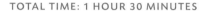

CRUST

1½ teaspoons flax meal

1 tablespoon water

2½ cups walnut pieces

¼ teaspoon sea salt

2 tablespoons coconut oil

2 tablespoons maple syrup

FILLING

4 large apples, peeled and thinly sliced

3 tablespoons maple syrup

3 tablespoons orange juice

½ teaspoon ground cinnamon

Preheat the oven to 375°F. Lightly oil the bottom and sides of a 9" tart pan with a removable bottom or a 9" pie plate.

To make the crust: In a small bowl, combine the flax meal and water, stir well, and set aside for 10 minutes to form a gel.

In a food processor, combine the walnuts and salt. Process until sandy. Add the oil, maple syrup, and reserved flax mixture and pulse to combine. Press the crust mixture into the bottom and up the sides of the pan. Bake for 12 to 15 minutes, or until the edges are golden brown. Let the crust cool for at least 10 minutes.

To make the filling: In a large bowl, toss the apples with the maple syrup, orange juice, and cinnamon to coat. Lift the apple slices from the syrup and reserve both the apples and the syrup.

Arrange the apples in concentric circles in the prebaked crust and bake for 30 minutes. Cover the tart with foil and bake for an additional 20 to 25 minutes, or until the apples are tender. Meanwhile, in a small saucepan over medium heat, heat the reserved syrup until it reduces to 3 tablespoons or a light syrup. Drizzle the syrup over the hot apples. Let the tart cool just until warm or chill (if desired).

Makes 6 servings

No-Bake Mini Lemon "Cheesecakes"

When you have a craving for lush, lemony cheesecake, give this treat a try. The surprise is that these mini-bites don't contain any dairy! The filling gets its creamy texture from the pine nuts, which need to be soaked in water for at least 4 hours.

TOTAL TIME: 30 MINUTES + CHILLING TIME

1 cup Grain-Free Granola (page 73) or wheat-free, gluten-free cinnamon-raisin granola

2 teaspoons coconut palm sugar

4 tablespoons coconut oil, divided

1 cup pine nuts, soaked in cool water for 4 to 8 hours

2 tablespoons + 2 teaspoons lemon juice

2 tablespoons + 1 teaspoon raw agave syrup

½ teaspoon grated lemon peel

Pinch of sea salt

1 cup blueberries or raspberries

Line 6 muffin cups or custard cups with paper liners.

In a mini food processor or blender, combine the granola and sugar. Process or blend until finely ground. Add 1 tablespoon of the coconut oil and process until the mixture begins to cling together. Press 1 tablespoon of the mixture in the bottom of each muffin cup and refrigerate for at least 30 minutes.

Rinse the food processor or blender. Drain the pine nuts. In the food processor or blender, combine the pine nuts, lemon juice, and agave syrup. Process until very smooth, scraping the sides of the processor or blender a few times as needed. Add the lemon peel, salt, and remaining 3 tablespoons coconut oil and process or blend until well mixed. Spoon into the muffin cups on top of the crust and top with the berries. Cover with plastic wrap and refrigerate for at least 3 hours, or until firm.

Makes 6 mini cheesecakes

Oatmeal-Raisin Cookies

Oatmeal cookies generously studded with dark raisins are an American classic. Baking the cookies at 2 different temperatures lets them spread at the lower temp and then bake to a delightful chewiness at the higher one.

TOTAL TIME: 55 MINUTES

    1 tablespoon chia seeds

    3 tablespoons water

    ½ cup almond butter

    ½ cup coconut palm sugar

    3 tablespoons coconut oil

    1½ teaspoons vanilla extract

    1⅓ cups gluten-free rolled oats

    1½ teaspoons ground cinnamon

    ½ teaspoon gluten-free baking powder

    ¼ teaspoon baking soda

    ¼ teaspoon sea salt

    ½ cup raisins

Preheat the oven to 275°F. Line 2 baking sheets with parchment paper.

In a small bowl, mix together the chia seeds and water and set aside for 15 minutes to form a gel.

In a large bowl, combine the almond butter, sugar, oil, and vanilla and beat with an electric mixer on medium speed for 2 minutes. Add the oats, cinnamon, baking powder, baking soda, salt, and reserved chia mixture and beat well. Stir in the raisins.

Drop golf ball–size balls of dough on the baking sheets, leaving several inches between each ball. They do spread. Bake for 9 minutes. Increase the heat to 350°F and bake for 14 minutes, or until the cookies are firm. Cool on the baking sheets for 5 to 10 minutes to firm up. Remove the cookies to racks to cool completely.

Makes 12 cookies

Triple Chocolate Brownies

Chocolate is my go-to indulgence. These brownies are so satisfying because they get triple deliciousness from cocoa, chocolate chips, and unsweetened chocolate.

TOTAL TIME: 35 MINUTES + COOLING TIME

2 tablespoons flax meal

6 tablespoons water

7 tablespoons coconut flour

¼ cup unsweetened cocoa powder

½ teaspoon sea salt

¼ teaspoon baking soda

½ cup coconut oil

1¼ cups gluten-free dark chocolate chips, divided

2 ounces high-quality gluten-free unsweetened chocolate, coarsely chopped

½ cup honey

1 teaspoon vanilla extract

Preheat the oven to 350°F. Line the bottom of an 8" × 8" baking pan with parchment paper and lightly oil the sides of the pan.

In a small bowl, combine the flax meal and water, stir well, and set aside for 10 minutes to thicken.

In a mixing bowl, combine the coconut flour, cocoa, salt, and baking soda. Whisk until well mixed.

In a small saucepan over low heat, heat the oil, 1 cup of the chocolate chips, and the chopped chocolate, stirring constantly, until the chocolate melts. Remove the pan from the heat and stir in the honey and vanilla. Add the reserved flax mixture and whisk to mix thoroughly. Pour into the dry ingredients and mix well. Pour the batter into the pan and sprinkle with the remaining ¼ cup chocolate chips. Bake for 15 minutes, or until a wooden pick inserted in the center of the brownies comes out slightly sticky. Cool in the pan on a rack for at least 15 minutes before cutting.

Makes approximately 12 brownies

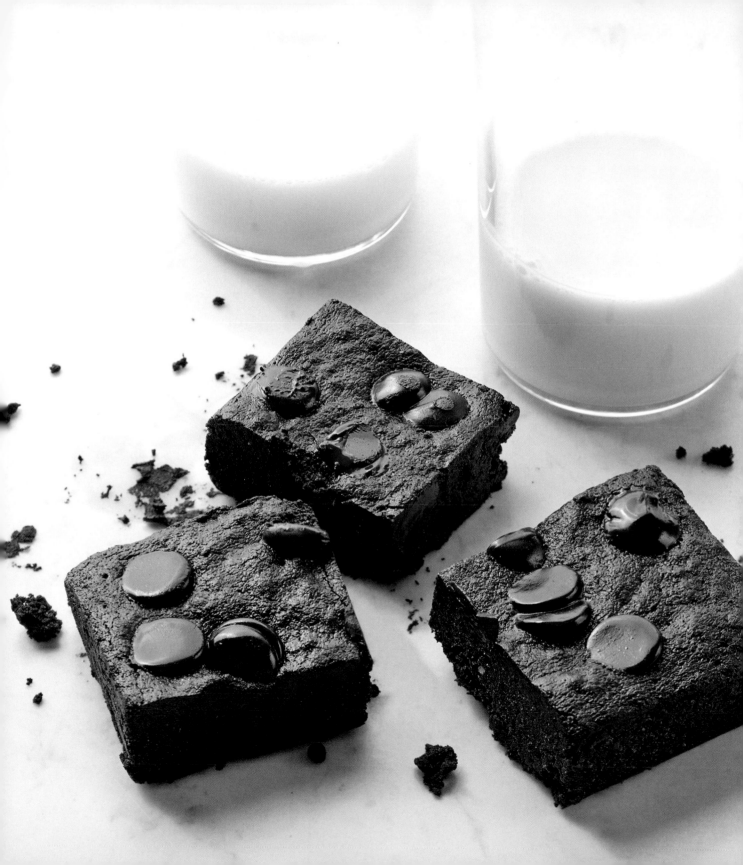

Peach-Cherry Cobbler

A cobbler is a deep-dish fruit pie with a crust on the top and fruit filling on the bottom, but no crust underneath. The colorful combination of pale peaches and bright red cherries peeks through the topping once the cobbler is baked.

TOTAL TIME: 30 MINUTES

4 large peaches, sliced with skin on

1 package (12 ounces) frozen dark sweet cherries, thawed and drained (1½ cups)

3 tablespoons honey, divided

4 teaspoons cornstarch

½ teaspoon ground ginger

¾ teaspoon ground cinnamon, divided

¾ cup gluten-free oat flour

¾ cup almond flour

1 teaspoon gluten-free baking powder

1 large egg, lightly beaten

3 tablespoons melted coconut oil

Preheat the oven to 375°F.

In an 8" × 8" baking dish, combine the peaches, cherries, and 1 tablespoon of the honey. Sprinkle with the cornstarch, ginger, and ¼ teaspoon of the cinnamon. Toss gently to blend the cornstarch with the fruit.

In a medium bowl, whisk together the oat flour, almond flour, baking powder, and remaining ½ teaspoon cinnamon. Add the egg, oil, and remaining 2 tablespoons honey and mix well. Spread the topping over the fruit. (It will not cover it completely.) Bake for 20 minutes, or until bubbling and a wooden pick inserted in the topping comes out clean. Serve warm.

Makes 6 servings

Pineapple Bars

Bar cookies make great snacks for lunch boxes or after-school treats. These are made with pineapple and sweetened with honey, a change from other bar cookies.

TOTAL TIME: 1 HOUR + CHILLING TIME

½ **cup gluten-free oat flour**

½ **cup almond flour**

3 **tablespoons coconut oil**

4 **tablespoons honey, divided**

⅛ **teaspoon sea salt**

1 **can (21 ounces) crushed pineapple in juice (do not drain)**

2 **tablespoons cornstarch**

3 **large eggs**

1 **teaspoon grated orange zest**

Preheat the oven to 350°F. Line an 8" × 8" baking pan with parchment paper, leaving an overhang on 2 opposite sides.

In a mini food processor, combine the oat flour, almond flour, oil, 1 tablespoon of the honey, and salt. Process until the mixture begins to stick together. Press into the bottom of the baking pan and bake for 10 to 15 minutes, or until partially baked and golden brown.

In a medium bowl, mix the pineapple and cornstarch. Add the eggs, orange zest, and remaining 3 tablespoons honey and mix well. Carefully pour over the partially baked crust and bake for 35 to 45 minutes, or until a small knife inserted near the center of the pan comes out clean. Cool in the pan on a rack. Refrigerate for 2 to 3 hours. Cut into bars.

Makes approximately 9 bars

Cherry-Almond Bars

These bars are flavored with raw almonds and dried cherries as well as a generous amount of coconut.

TOTAL TIME: 45 MINUTES

3 tablespoons ground flax meal

½ cup + 1 tablespoon water

2 cups whole raw almonds

1 cup juice-sweetened dried cherries

1 cup shredded unsweetened coconut

1 teaspoon grated orange peel

½ teaspoon baking soda

¼ teaspoon sea salt

¼ cup orange juice

¾ teaspoon almond extract

Preheat the oven to 350°F. Lightly oil an 11" × 7" baking dish.

In a small bowl, mix the flax meal with the water and set aside for 10 minutes, or until a gel forms.

In a food processor, combine the almonds and cherries. Process until finely ground. Add the coconut, orange peel, baking soda, and salt and process until thoroughly mixed. Add the reserved flax mixture, orange juice, and almond extract and process until the dough is thoroughly mixed.

Spread the dough in the baking dish. The mixture will be sticky. Bake for 20 to 25 minutes, or until a wooden pick inserted in the center comes out clean. Cool in the pan on a rack. Cut into squares and serve.

Makes approximately 15 bars

Maple-Pecan Blender Ice Cream

Yes, it's possible to make ice cream without an ice cream maker, as you'll discover when you try this irresistible recipe. Just make sure to use a high-speed blender (1,000 watts or more). I like to make it with dark, amber-colored maple syrup because its flavor is stronger than lighter maple syrup. If you can't find the dark syrup, use what is available, but make sure it's pure maple syrup.

TOTAL TIME: 1 HOUR

6 tablespoons dark amber pure maple syrup

¼ cup full-fat, canned coconut milk

¼ teaspoon sea salt

1⅔ cups coarsely chopped pecan pieces, divided

3 cups large ice cubes

In a high-speed blender, combine the syrup, coconut milk, and salt. Add 1⅓ cups of the pecans and the ice cubes and blend on the "ice cream" setting, or begin on low and increase the speed to high until the mixture is smooth and thick. Scrape down the sides of the blender as needed. If the mixture is too thin, add more ice cubes. Stir in the remaining ⅓ cup pecans and serve immediately.

For a firmer texture, scrape the ice cream into a freezer-safe container and freeze for 30 to 40 minutes. Store in the covered container in the freezer. Remove from the freezer about 10 to 15 minutes before serving to soften.

Makes 6 servings

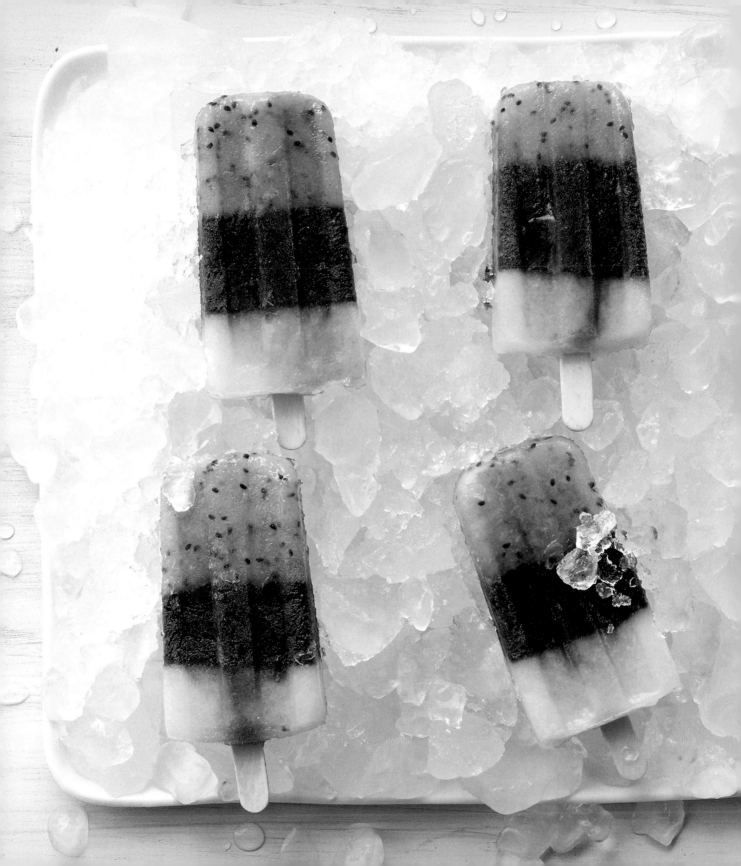

Frozen Fruit Pops

If my kids had their way, the freezer would be stocked only with ice cream. This refreshing dessert allows me to give them (and myself) a healthy, sweet treat.

TOTAL TIME: 15 MINUTES + FREEZING TIME

 2 large kiwifruit, peeled

¼ teaspoon grated lime peel

 1 cup frozen pitted sweet cherries, thawed

⅛ teaspoon almond extract

¾ cup cubed fresh or canned and drained pineapple

⅛ teaspoon grated orange peel

In a mini blender, puree the kiwi until smooth. Transfer ¾ cup of the mixture to a glass measuring cup (discard any excess or reserve for another use), add the lime peel, and stir to mix. Pour into 6 molds (4 ounces each) and freeze for at least 1 hour or until almost solid. The puree will not fill the molds.

Rinse out the blender canister. Puree the cherries and almond extract until smooth. Pour over the kiwi layer. The cherry puree will not top off the mold. Insert a wooden fruit pop stick into each mold. Freeze for 45 minutes or until almost solid.

Rinse out the blender canister. Blend the pineapple and orange peel until smooth. Pour over the cherry layer to come nearly to the top of the molds. Freeze pops for several hours or until solid. Before serving, dip the molds briefly in warm water to loosen the pops.

Makes 6 servings

Warm Chocolate-Almond Dip

When I was testing the desserts in this book with family and friends, this simple-to-make dip was a surprise favorite. The chocolate dip has the perfect amount of almond flavor. Pair the dip with slices of your favorite fruits.

TOTAL TIME: 15 MINUTES

¼ **cup creamy almond butter**

¼ **cup unsweetened almond milk**

3 **tablespoons honey**

1 **ounce gluten-free unsweetened chocolate, broken into pieces**

⅛ **teaspoon almond extract**

Pinch of sea salt

Fresh fruit, such as strawberries, sliced pears, and bananas

In a small saucepan over medium-low heat, cook the almond butter, almond milk, and honey, stirring constantly, for 3 minutes, or until heated through and smooth. Remove from the heat and stir in the chocolate, almond extract, and salt until smooth.

Serve the warm dip with fresh fruit. Cover and refrigerate any leftovers and reheat before serving. If needed to achieve the desired consistency, add a little more almond milk when reheating.

Makes 10 servings

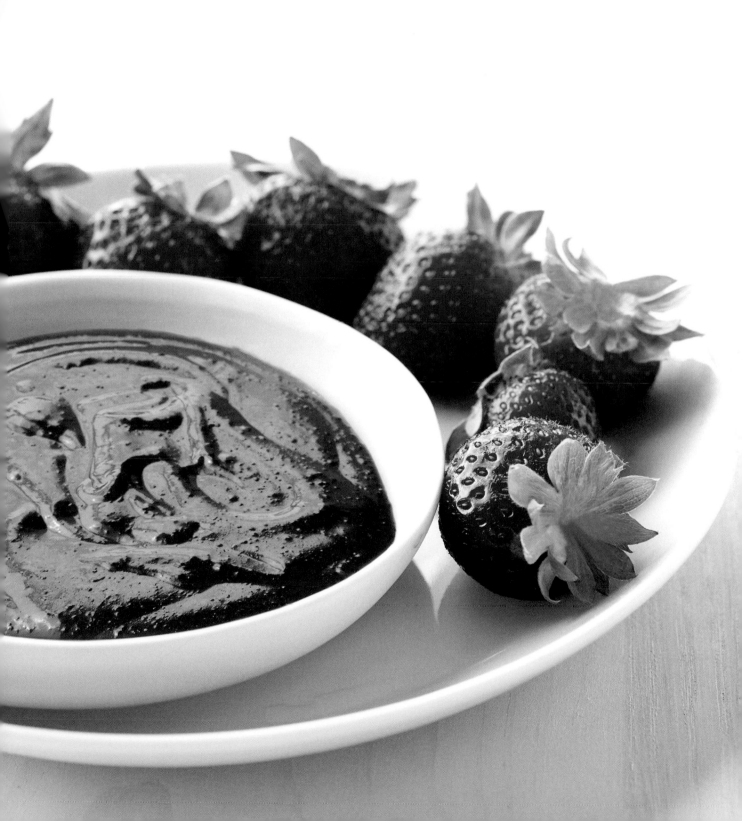

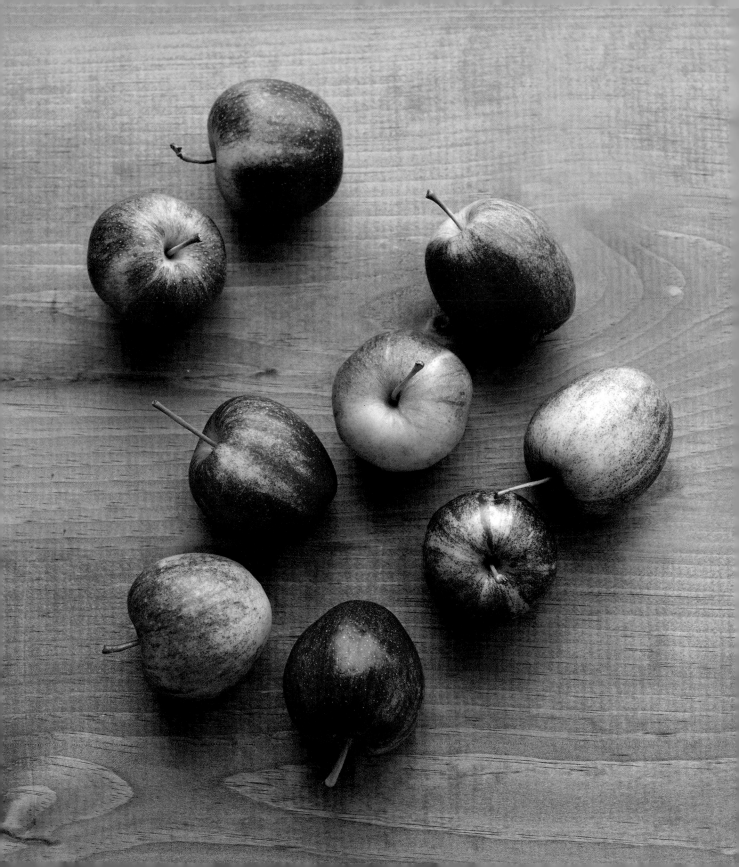

a final word

I'm passionate about helping people eat a cleaner diet and lose weight. As I explained in the introduction, I know what it's like to be overweight. I also know how great it feels to lose those excess pounds, keep them off, and become healthy. I want *The Healthy You Diet* to inspire and encourage you to take advantage of all of the possibilities that life has to offer.

One of the most important things I hope you take away from this book is the need to believe in yourself. Believe that you can take the first steps by eliminating certain foods from your diet. Believe that you can stay with the 14-day program and you'll be amazed with the results. Believe that you will lose weight, feel better, look better, sleep better, think more clearly, and have boundless energy. If you believe it, you can do it.

If you need extra motivation or additional support, then I suggest that you sign up for the online Healthy You Diet challenge. Every few months, I offer a free 14-day program online. Thousands of people—people just like you—sign up, and everyone works together to lose weight and remain motivated. I'll personally guide you, using Facebook and Twitter, to help you reach your goals. I'll be available to answer questions and provide support, encouragement, and motivation. During the 14-day challenge, you'll receive positive encouragement and support from thousands of other men and women who are also eager to eat better and lose weight. You'll have the opportunity to share your experience and encourage others on the program. Those who participated in the 14-day challenges have lost anywhere from 6 to 14 pounds in just 2 weeks. If you decide to sign up for the challenge online, use this book as the perfect resource for cooking along with the challenge.

To join me on an upcoming challenge, go to healthyyouchallenge.com or healthyyoudiet.com.

If you don't want to take my word for how successful the 14-day challenge is, then read what other participants have said.

Kristy O:
"Wow! I just weighed myself, and I am down 7 pounds in 1 week! This program rocks!"

Mary H:
"Since starting the diet, I've lost 16 pounds and feel 10 years younger."

Melissa M:
"I'm down 5 pounds in the first week. But moreover, I am shocked at the changes in my body and skin. I feel great!"

Kathy S:
"I lost 4 pounds in just 4 days! I wish I had known about this process a long time ago. Thank you, thank you, thank you. I feel like I have my own personal weight-loss coach."

Kelly B:
"I lost 6 pounds in the first week of the program! My appetite has dramatically reduced, and my sugar and salt cravings are gone!"

Changing your eating habits, especially if your current diet includes unhealthy fast food or highly processed convenience foods, is challenging. But it's necessary for your health and well-being. With that in mind, I made sure that all the meals I created for the 14-day Healthy You Diet program are quick and simple to make. Will you feel deprived? No! Will you wonder how food can be so flavorful and so good for you? Absolutely yes!

With a business to run and two small kids to run after, I know that shopping for food and preparing meals takes time and effort. That's why the recipes in this cookbook include user-friendly, readily available ingredients and simple techniques to get meals on the table as quickly as possible. These recipes are ideal for your entire family. I know, because I serve these dishes to my family every day. Let me know how you enjoy them.

The knowledge, inspiration, and encouragement you need to take action, lose weight, and lead a healthy life are all right here in *The Healthy You Diet*.

appendix a meal plans

Elimination Phase (Days 1–7)

	DAY 1	DAY 2	DAY 3	DAY 4	DAY 5	DAY 6	DAY 7
Breakfast	Very Berry Smoothie (page 96)	Oatmeal with Fresh Berries and Almond Milk (page 74)	Super Green Juice (page 97)	Vegetable Scramble (page 79) and Oatmeal (page 74)	Radiant Red Juice (page 98)	Vegetable Omelet (page 78) and 1 slice melon	Spinach, Tomato, and Basil Frittata (page 77) or Vegetable Omelet (page 78) and ½ cup fresh fruit
Lunch	Turkey and Avocado Sandwich (page 121)	Strawberry–Goat Cheese Salad (page 145)	Three-Bean Salad (page 136)	Grilled Salmon and Citrus Salad (page 151)	Vegetarian Chili (page 118)	Pasta Salad with Vegetables (page 138)	Quinoa, Cranberry, and Almond Salad (page 139)
Snack	1 oz low-fat string cheese and 1 medium apple	5–6 oz Greek yogurt (nonfat, sugar-free) and 10 raw almonds	1 pear or apple	Strawberry-Banana Smoothie (page 95)	Sliced banana and 4-6 strawberries	1 apple and 1 Tbsp natural peanut butter	Hummus with Vegetables (page 201)
Dinner	Grilled Herb Chicken (page 167), steamed broccoli, and green salad	Chicken and Vegetable Stir-Fry (page 169)	Miso-Glazed Salmon with Bok Choy (page 173)	Pasta Primavera (page 187)	Flank Steak with Arugula (page 184) and 6 oz red or white wine (optional)	Halibut with Tomato-Mango Salsa (page 179), quinoa, steamed asparagus, and 6 oz red or white wine (optional)	Chicken Tacos (page 172)
Eliminated Items	Sugar	Wheat (plus sugar)	Dairy (plus sugar and wheat)	Highly processed foods (plus sugar, wheat, and dairy)	Artificial sweeteners (plus sugar, wheat, dairy, and highly processed foods)	Red meat (plus sugar, wheat, dairy, highly processed foods, and artificial sweeteners)	Alcohol (plus sugar, wheat, dairy, highly processed foods, artificial sweeteners, and red meat)

Clean Phase (Days 8–14)

	DAY 8	DAY 9	DAY 10	DAY 11	DAY 12	DAY 13	DAY 14
Breakfast	Super Green Juice (page 97)	Pineapple-Avocado Smoothie (page 91)	Strawberry-Banana Smoothie (page 95)	Vegetable Scramble (page 79) and Oatmeal (page 74)	Radiant Red Juice (page 98)	Vegetable Omelet (page 78) and 1 cup fresh fruit	Super Green Juice (page 97)
Lunch	Red Quinoa Salad with Black Beans and Avocado (page 141)	Vegetable Soup (page 113) and green salad	Lentil-Carrot Salad (page 137)	Spinach, Pear, and Walnut Salad (page 157)	Chicken and Brussels Sprouts Slaw (page 148)	Wild Rice–Spinach Soup (page 104)	Crab, Mango, and Avocado Stacks (page 152)
Snack	Fresh Salsa and Tortilla Chips (page 204)	Celery sticks and 1 Tbsp natural peanut butter	1 cup red or green grapes	Magic Mango Smoothie (page 90)	1 apple and 10 raw almonds	Hummus with Vegetables (page 201)	1 apple or pear
Dinner	Crab Cakes (page 195) and steamed green beans	Black Bean Tostadas with Salsa (page 197)	Rosemary Chicken and Wild Rice (page 166)	Fish Tacos with Mango-Avocado Salsa (page 180)	Seared Scallops and Succotash (page 183)	Chicken Skewers with Honey-Lime-Chile Sauce (page 171) and green salad	Snapper and Asparagus en Papillote (page 174) and brown basmati rice
Eliminated Items	Sugar, wheat, dairy, highly processed foods, artificial sweeteners, red meat, and alcohol	Sugar, wheat, dairy, highly processed foods, artificial sweeteners, red meat, and alcohol	Sugar, wheat, dairy, highly processed foods, artificial sweeteners, red meat, and alcohol	Sugar, wheat, dairy, highly processed foods, artificial sweeteners, red meat, and alcohol	Sugar, wheat, dairy, highly processed foods, artificial sweeteners, red meat, and alcohol	Sugar, wheat, dairy, highly processed foods, artificial sweeteners, red meat, and alcohol	Sugar, wheat, dairy, highly processed foods, artificial sweeteners, red meat, and alcohol

appendix b

shopping lists

Thanks to the detailed daily meal plans that I created for the Healthy You Diet, you don't have to make choices about what to eat during the 2-week program. Once you finish the program, I encourage you to follow the Healthy You approach to food: Eat clean food, avoid the Big Seven, and maintain controlled portions. If you do so, you will lose more weight and reach your target goal, all while enjoying delicious, healthy food. You can also stay on the Clean Phase for as long as you like. For additional variety once you're finished with the 14-day program, you can substitute any of the Healthy You recipes in this book for those in the 14-day meal plans.

The shopping lists below—one for Week 1 and one for Week 2—will help you plan for the 14-day program. Don't be discouraged by the number of items. Many of them are everyday staples like salt, pepper, olive oil, and Dijon mustard, which you probably have on hand. I've made sure that the lists include everything you need, so you don't have to make repeat trips to the grocery store.

You will notice that I don't include how much of each item you should purchase. I assume that you will be preparing different numbers of portions, depending on how many people you are cooking for. The lists are merely a guide to help you stock your pantry.

You can always double a recipe and enjoy it the next day. For example, you can prepare and eat Three-Bean Salad (page 136) for Day 3's lunch instead of making Grilled Salmon and Citrus Salad (page 151) on Day 4. If, however, you do have the time to make every recipe on the 14-day program, I encourage you to do so, as you just may find some new favorites.

The Healthy You Diet: Week 1 Shopping List

FRUITS

Apples (red and green)

Avocados (Hass)

Bananas

Berries (blueberries, raspberries, strawberries)

Cranberries (dried, juice-sweetened)

Grapefruit

Kalamata olives (optional)

Kiwifruit (optional for fruit salad)

Lemons

Limes

Mango

Melon (cantaloupe, honeydew, or watermelon)

Oranges (navel and Valencias for juice)

Pear (optional)

Pineapple (optional for fruit salad)

Tomatoes (regular and plum)

VEGETABLES AND FRESH HERBS

Arugula

Asparagus

Baby spinach

Bean sprouts

Belgian endive (optional)

Bell peppers (red or yellow)

Bok choy

Broccoli

Carrots

Celery

Cucumbers

Eggplant

Fennel bulb (optional)

Garlic

Kale

Mushrooms (cremini)

Onions (red and yellow)

Romaine lettuce

Scallions

Shallots

Snap or snow peas

Yellow squash

Zucchini

Basil

Cilantro

Ginger

Parsley (flat-leaf)

Rosemary

Thyme (or dried)

POULTRY, EGGS, MEAT, AND FISH

Boneless, skinless
chicken breasts

Eggs

Flank steak

Halibut or cod
fillets

Salmon fillets

Turkey breast
(sliced)

DAIRY

Goat cheese, fresh

Greek yogurt,
plain (nonfat,
sugar-free)

String cheese
(low-fat)

BREADS

Corn tortillas
(soft)

Whole wheat,
whole grain, or
sourdough
bread (only 2
slices on Day 1)

DRINKS

Almond milk
(unsweetened,
plain)

RICE, PASTA, GRAINS, AND BEANS

Black beans
(canned)

Brown rice

Brown rice pasta
(fettuccine,
shells, or fusilli)

Chickpeas
(canned)

Kidney beans
(canned)

Oats (gluten-free,
steel-cut)

Quinoa

White beans, such
as Northern,
navy, or
cannellini
(canned)

SPICES AND CONDIMENTS

Chicken broth (low-sodium)

Chili powder

Chipotle chile peppers in adobo

Cocoa powder (unsweetened)

Coriander (ground)

Crushed red-pepper flakes (optional)

Cumin (ground)

Dijon mustard

Garlic powder

Honey

Hot sauce (optional)

Italian seasoning blend

Miso paste (white or yellow)

Onion powder

Oregano

Paprika

Peanut butter (natural, no sugar added)

Pepper, ground, black

Sea salt

Soy sauce (gluten-free, reduced-sodium) or tamari

Spicy mustard (optional)

Tahini

Vegetable broth (low-sodium)

NUTS AND SEEDS

Almonds

Pecans

Sesame seeds (black)

OILS AND VINEGARS

Balsamic vinegar (red and white)

Extra-virgin olive oil

Peanut oil

Red wine vinegar

Rice vinegar (or mirin)

Vegetable oil

The Healthy You Diet: Week 2 Shopping List

FRUITS

Apples (green and Granny Smith or Fuji)

Avocados (Hass)

Bananas

Berries (blueberries, raspberries, strawberries)

Grapes (red or green)

Lemons

Limes

Mango

Oranges (Valencias for juice)

Pears

Pineapple

Pomegranate seeds or juice-sweetened dried cherries

Raisins (no sugar added)

Tomatoes (regular and cherry)

VEGETABLES AND FRESH HERBS

Arugula

Asparagus

Baby spinach

Belgian endive

Bell peppers (red and, if desired, green and yellow)

Brussels sprouts

Cabbage

Carrots

Cauliflower

Celery

Chives

Corn (fresh, frozen, or canned)

Cucumbers

Fennel bulb

Garlic

Green beans

Jalapeño chile peppers

Kale

Leeks

Lettuce (spring salad mix)

Mushrooms (cremini or button)

Onions (red and yellow)

Romaine

Scallions

Shallots

Zucchini

Cilantro

Dill (or dried)

Ginger

Parsley (flat-leaf)

Rosemary

Thyme (or dried)

POULTRY, EGGS, AND SEAFOOD

- Boneless, skinless chicken breasts
- Cod fillets or mahi-mahi
- Crabmeat (lump)
- Eggs
- Rotisserie chicken
- Sea scallops
- Snapper or halibut fillets

BREAD

- Corn tortillas (soft)

DRINKS

- Almond milk (unsweetened, plain)

SPICES AND CONDIMENTS

- Agave nectar (or honey)
- Bay leaves
- Chives
- Crab-boil seasoning
- Dijon mustard
- Honey
- Hot sauce
- Maple syrup (pure)
- Oat flour
- Paprika (optional)
- Peanut butter (natural, no sugar added)
- Pepper (ground, black and white)
- Red-pepper flakes
- Sambal oelek
- Sea salt
- Soy sauce (gluten-free, reduced-sodium) or tamari
- Tahini
- Tomatoes (canned, diced, and fire-roasted)
- Vegetable broth (low-sodium)

GRAINS AND BEANS

Black beans (canned)

Brown basmati rice

Chickpeas (canned)

Edamame (or baby lima)

Lentils (green or brown)

Oats (gluten-free, steel-cut)

Quinoa

Red quinoa

Wild rice

NUTS

Almonds

Hazelnuts

Walnuts

OILS AND VINEGARS

Cider vinegar

Extra-virgin olive oil

Hazelnut oil

Peanut oil

Red wine vinegar

appendix c

keeping a food journal

On June 15, 2005, I drank a green juice for breakfast, ate a three-bean salad with homemade tortilla chips for lunch, munched some trail mix for an afternoon snack, and enjoyed agave-glazed salmon, brown rice, and snow peas for dinner. All these years later, I can still recall that information. I have no idea what I wore that day, what happened at work, or what the weather was like, but I do know what I ate. Why? Because I recorded everything I ate in a food journal.

Journals have been shown to be a key tool for weight-loss success. A study performed by researchers from Kaiser Permanente Center for Health Research found that keeping a food diary was the number one predictor of weight loss in their study participants—higher on the list than age, body mass index, or even exercise habits!

Some people view journaling as a burden—yet another nagging task on the daily to-do list. But I've found that this record-keeping practice yields positive results. When you write down what you eat and drink, how much, and when, you become much more aware of the food choices you make throughout the day.

There are many different ways to keep a food journal. Tuck a small notebook and a pen into your purse or backpack or use a food-tracking program on your computer or smartphone. I've included this 14-day journal to get you started.

ELIMINATION PHASE

DATE:_____ MORNING WEIGHT (OPTIONAL): _____

	TIME	MEAL DESCRIPTION	OTHER NOTES
Breakfast			
Lunch			
Snack			
Dinner			

ELIMINATION PHASE

DATE:_____MORNING WEIGHT (OPTIONAL): _____

	TIME	MEAL DESCRIPTION	OTHER NOTES
Breakfast			
Lunch			
Snack			
Dinner			

ELIMINATION PHASE

DATE:_____ MORNING WEIGHT (OPTIONAL): _____

	TIME	MEAL DESCRIPTION	OTHER NOTES
Breakfast			
Lunch			
Snack			
Dinner			

ELIMINATION PHASE

DATE:_____ MORNING WEIGHT (OPTIONAL): _____

	TIME	MEAL DESCRIPTION	OTHER NOTES
Breakfast			
Lunch			
Snack			
Dinner			

ELIMINATION PHASE

DATE:_____ MORNING WEIGHT (OPTIONAL): _____

	TIME	MEAL DESCRIPTION	OTHER NOTES
Breakfast			
Lunch			
Snack			
Dinner			

ELIMINATION PHASE

DATE:_____ MORNING WEIGHT (OPTIONAL): _____

	TIME	MEAL DESCRIPTION	OTHER NOTES
Breakfast			
Lunch			
Snack			
Dinner			

ELIMINATION PHASE

DATE:_____ MORNING WEIGHT (OPTIONAL): _____

	TIME	MEAL DESCRIPTION	OTHER NOTES
Breakfast			
Lunch			
Snack			
Dinner			

CLEAN PHASE

DATE:_____ MORNING WEIGHT (OPTIONAL): _____

	TIME	MEAL DESCRIPTION	OTHER NOTES
Breakfast			
Lunch			
Snack			
Dinner			

CLEAN PHASE

DATE:_____ MORNING WEIGHT (OPTIONAL): _____

	TIME	MEAL DESCRIPTION	OTHER NOTES
Breakfast			
Lunch			
Snack			
Dinner			

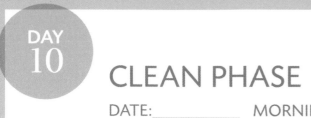

CLEAN PHASE

DATE:_____ MORNING WEIGHT (OPTIONAL): _____

	TIME	MEAL DESCRIPTION	OTHER NOTES
Breakfast			
Lunch			
Snack			
Dinner			

CLEAN PHASE

DATE:_____ MORNING WEIGHT (OPTIONAL): _____

	TIME	MEAL DESCRIPTION	OTHER NOTES
Breakfast			
Lunch			
Snack			
Dinner			

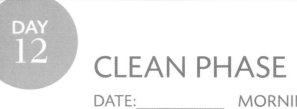

CLEAN PHASE

DATE:_____ MORNING WEIGHT (OPTIONAL): _____

	TIME	MEAL DESCRIPTION	OTHER NOTES
Breakfast			
Lunch			
Snack			
Dinner			

CLEAN PHASE

DATE:_____ MORNING WEIGHT (OPTIONAL): _____

	TIME	MEAL DESCRIPTION	OTHER NOTES
Breakfast			
Lunch			
Snack			
Dinner			

CLEAN PHASE

DATE:_____ MORNING WEIGHT (OPTIONAL): _____

	TIME	MEAL DESCRIPTION	OTHER NOTES
Breakfast			
Lunch			
Snack			
Dinner			

acknowledgments

So many people were instrumental in making this book a reality.

To my children, Kaelie and Luke, who are just starting to understand how important it is to follow your dreams and be passionate about something. I love their simple explanation of what I do: "My mommy helps people eat healthy food."

To my husband, Matt Dieter, for being my most enthusiastic cheerleader and believing in my dreams.

To my sister, Michele; my parents, Bob and Louise; and my in-laws, Barbara, Don, Di, and Holly, for always being my passionate supporters and constantly cheering me on.

To my good friend and colleague, Ellen Madden: Having you by my side for the past 7 years has made every step of the way so much more fun. Who would have guessed that one of my best interns would become my most valued business partner? Every day, I feel thankful for your continued hard work, your encouragement, and your support.

I also want to thank Cindy Ratzlaff. It was your introductions that made this dream come true. I am so fortunate to have met you. I look forward to working with you on all my future projects. Your advice and knowledge are invaluable.

To my agent, Stephanie Tade, for believing in me and this project and for making it all happen.

To Harriet Bell: I couldn't have done this without you. You are such a talented writer and editor. I want to thank you for all the long hours and hard work you put in to help me make this book come to fruition.

To Matt Kadey, Rochelle Schmidt, Lori Powell, Katherine Hamlin, and Edward Gallagher for your invaluable expertise when it comes to recipe development, recipe testing, food styling, and prop styling. And to Brandi Hopstein for helping me look my best on camera—makeup is definitely an art form I need help with.

This book wouldn't have been possible without the incredible team at Rodale Books: Maria Rodale, Mary Ann Naples, Jennifer Lang Levesque, Jeff Batzli, Carol Angstadt, Amy King, Mitch Mandel, Troy Schnyder, Emily Weber, Kristin Kiser, Hope Clarke, Evan Klonsky, Brent Gallenberger, and Mollie Grewe—and a very special thanks to my editor, Dervla Kelly. You have all been such a pleasure to work with. Thank you! I feel so fortunate to be part of the Rodale family.

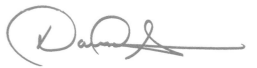

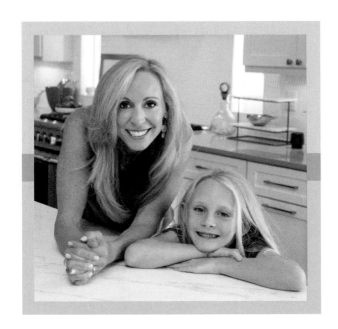

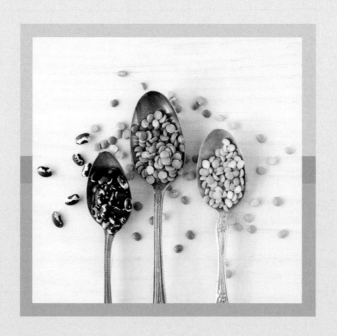

Index

Underscored page references indicate sidebars and tables. **Boldface** references indicate photographs.

Exercise
>for Almost Achiever diet personality, 11
>for Flip-Flopper diet personality, 9
>by Food Abusers, 10
>intense, calorie requirements and, 37
>for Nonbeliever diet personality, 8
>for Remote Controller diet personality, 7
>suggestions for, 49–50

F

Fish
>Fish Tacos with Mango-Avocado Salsa, 180, **181**
>Grilled Salmon and Citrus Salad, **150**, 151
>Halibut with Tomato-Mango Salsa, **178**, 179
>Miso-Glazed Salmon with Bok Choy, 173
>Sesame-Crusted Ahi Tuna and Cucumber-Seaweed Salad, 154, **155**
>Snapper and Asparagus en Papillote, 174, **175**
>Steamed Sole with Butternut Squash Puree, 176
>Tuna Niçoise Salad, 153

Flatbreads
>Mediterranean Flatbread Pizzas, 192–93, **193**

Flax meal, 58
Flip-Flopper diet personality, 9
Flour
>coconut, 57
>oat
>>Apple-Oat Bread, 85
>quinoa, 61–62

Food Abuser diet personality, 10, 12
Food allergies
>food substitutes and, 38
>wheat allergy, 16

Food journals, 7, 8, 9, 10, 11, 246
>for Clean Phase, 254–60
>for Elimination Phase, 247–53

Food shopping
>guidelines for, 10, 20–21, 21
>Week 1 list for, 239, 240–42
>Week 2 list for, 239, 243–45

Frittata
>Spinach, Tomato, and Basil Frittata, **76**, 77

Fruits. *See also specific fruits*
>Dirty Dozen and Clean Fifteen, 53
>Frozen Fruit Pops, **230**, 231
>organic, 53
>replacing processed foods with, 20

G

Garlic
>Garlic Shrimp Pasta with Roasted Tomatoes, 177
>Grilled Vegetable Wraps with Roasted Garlic Bean Spread, **122**, 123

Gazpacho
>Roasted Vegetable and Strawberry Gazpacho, 115

Ghrelin, 48
Gluten, 16, 17
Goal setting, 9
Goat cheese
>Strawberry–Goat Cheese Salad, 145, **145**

Granola
>Cranberry-Orange Granola, 72
>Grain-Free Granola, 73

Grapefruit
>Grilled Salmon and Citrus Salad, **150**, 151

Green beans
>Tuna Niçoise Salad, 153
>Vegetable Soup, 113

Greens, cleaning, 143
Grill pan, for cooking chicken, 168
Guacamole, 200
Guilt, postindulgence, 43

H

Halibut
>Halibut with Tomato-Mango Salsa, **178**, 179

Hazelnuts
>Maple-Hazelnut Vinaigrette, 160, **160**

Headaches
>after artificial sweetener elimination, 36, 38
>after sugar elimination, 38
>from unstable blood sugar, 14
>from wheat allergy, 16